*The Practical Guide to the
Genetic Family History*

The Practical Guide to the Genetic Family History

Robin L. Bennett

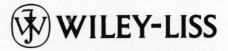

WILEY-LISS

A JOHN WILEY & SONS, INC., PUBLICATION

New York • Chichester • Weinheim • Brisbane • Singapore • Toronto

Library of Congress Cataloging in Publication Data:

Bennett, Robin, MS, CGC.
    The practical guide to the genetic family history / by Robin
Bennett.
        p.   cm.
    Includes index.
    ISBN 0-471-25154-2 (pbk. : alk. paper)
    1. Genetic counseling.   2. Medical history taking.   3. Geneology.
I. Title.
RB155.7.B46   1999
616'.042—dc21   98-37273

Printed in the United States of America.

10 9 8 7 6 5 4 3 2

To Scott, Mom, and Mr. Tougaw:
thanks for believing in me

CONTENTS

Illustrations and Tables

Foreword

Robin Bennett's book is a superb introduction to clinical approaches in medical genetics. Centered on the most traditional diagnostic tool in clinical genetics—the family history—she presents a well-balanced discussion of all of its aspects including the many applications for diagnosis of genetic disease. The book is based on extensive personal experience and provides much practical and useful information. But there is much more! The book's contents reflect the most recent genetic developments in all medical specialties, not just pediatric and obstetric aspects. Thus the rapidly expanding knowledge in cancer genetics is covered, as are various genetic considerations about assisted reproduction for women as well as for men (intracytoplasmic sperm injection). There are many helpful tables for a variety of potential genetic problems including hearing loss, mental retardation, dementia, seizures, and many others. A useful general chapter covers classical Mendelian patterns of inheritance as well as the relatively recently discovered mechanisms of genetic transmission such as imprinting and dynamic mutations.

Unlike in many books on medical genetics there is emphasis on the personal and human side of dealing with patients and families at all times. Useful lists cite reference books with critical discussions of their content. Historical and personal vignettes enliven the text.

This volume will be an essential resource for every genetics clinic and will aid medical geneticists and genetic counselors, whether experienced or in training. In addition, this text will be very helpful for both primary care and specialist physicians and allied health professionals, as well as for students of medicine, nursing, midwifery, and genetic counseling who need an up to date reference that emphasizes both the science and art of modern clinical genetics.

I have worked with Robin Bennett side by side in our genetics clinic at the University of Washington Medical Center for 15 years. She is superb in helping patients, families, and her colleagues with a multitude of practical, logistical, psychological, and diagnostic problems. This book demonstrates that she is even better informed with excellent judgment in more areas then I had realized. We can be grateful that her wise counsel and up to date knowledge can now be shared with a wide community of professionals whose patients will greatly benefit from these insights.

ARNO G. MOTULSKY
Departments of Medicine and Genetics
University of Washington
Seattle, Washington

Preface

When I consider the changes that have occurred over the past 15 years of my career as a genetic counselor, I feel the excitement that Anthony van Leeuwenhoek must have experienced in the early 1700s when he discovered a whole new world by using lenses to study microscopic objects. The simple rules of Gregor Mendel are no longer sufficient to explain complex patterns of inheritance reflecting such fascinating phenomena as imprinting and mitochondrial inheritance (see Chapter 2). The distinction blurs between environmental and genetic factors in the expression of disease. Genes do not operate in a vacuum; they interact with each other and with the environmental milieu. We are at the cusp of the chasm in understanding these complex gene–environment interactions. Every specialist in health care needs a basic foundation in human genetics to be able to recognize inherited disorders and familial disease susceptibility in patients, and to provide them with appropriate medical care.

The gateway to recognizing inherited disorders in a patient is a thorough medical–family history recorded in the form of a pedigree. A pedigree can assist the clinician in medical diagnosis, deciding on testing strategies, identifying patterns of inheritance, calculating risks, determining reproductive options, distinguishing genetic from other risk factors, making decisions on medical management and surveillance, developing patient rapport, and patient education (see Chapter 1). A pedigree is an important component of the medical record.

Although most clinicians have a cursory knowledge of the symbols that are used in constructing a pedigree, many are unaware that a standard set of symbols was developed through a peer review process, by the Pedigree Standardization Task Force of the National Society of Genetic Counselors, and adopted by the medical genetics community as a system of nomenclature. Pedigrees are of little value if each clinician uses a unique system of nomenclature. Using the appropriate pedigree symbolization is important for correct interpretation of a pedigree.

My intent in writing this book is to provide clinicians not only with the "hows" of taking a medical–family history and recording a pedigree, but also the "whys." Pedigree nomenclature and the approach to recording a medical–family history are reviewed in Chapter 3. Chapter 4 may remind you of the "Cliff's Notes" you read in college to understand a classic tome of English literature. It is meant to provide a basic overview of the directed questions to ask when recording a medical-family history for a specific medical indication (e.g., renal disease, hearing loss, mental illness). I have not reviewed every medical system. My choice of disease categories is based on my experience of operating a toll-free genetic resource line for health care professionals; these are the categories of disease that I receive the most questions about. Because of the ever-growing importance of genetic susceptibility factors in cancer, Chapter 5 is devoted solely to this topic. Sample cases for practicing drawing pedigrees are provided in Appendix A.6.

Throughout the book I use clinical examples to illustrate certain themes. The case scenarios and pedigrees are based on hypothetical families. The names, family relationships, and psychosocial issues are fictitious, although the clinical information is often based on facts drawn from several families I have seen in my practice. The pedigrees of the Darwin–Wedgwood family (Figure 3.11) and of actress Elizabeth Taylor's immediate family (Figure 3.6) were drawn from information available in the public domain.

Pedigree analysis requires that the health facts recorded on individuals be accurate. This requires obtaining medical records on family members. Although this is often time consuming, it is necessary. Chapter 6 details how to assist a patient in obtaining medical records, including death certificates. There is also information about how patients can research their medical–family history and learn to record their own medical pedigree. It is helpful to the clinician if a patient has done the footwork in obtaining medical-family history information in advance of an appointment.

Adoption and assisted reproductive technologies using gamete donation provide challenges in taking a medical–family history (see Chapters 7 and 8, respectively). A model medical-family history form to be used for adoption is detailed in Appendix A.4. This form was developed by the Education Committee of the Council of Regional Genetics Networks (CORN). This form can easily be adapted for use by programs providing assisted reproductive technology services.

Genetic information carries unique personal, family, and social consequences. If a potential genetic disorder is identified through pedigree analysis, it is important that the patient and family members be referred to a board-certified genetic counselor or medical geneticist with the appropriate expertise. Information on how to find a genetic specialist in your geographic area, and what to expect from a genetic consultation, is given in Chapter 9.

Some of the numerous ethical issues to consider in recording a pedigree are detailed in Chapter 10. Researchers and individuals who are considering publishing a pedigree will find valuable information regarding issues to consider when involved in a family study or in publishing a case report.

This volume is meant to be a handy reference—a "Cliff's Notes" for making a genetic risk assessment, with a pedigree being the primary tool. To find more information about a specific condition, you will need to turn to one of the many excellent references on genetic disorders outlined in The Genetics Library (Appendix A.5). Any health care provider including physicians, nurses, medical social workers, and physician assistants will benefit from learning this approach to pedigree analysis.

Many people assisted me with the development of the ideas for this book as well as reviewing drafts of the manuscript. I am indebted to Robert Resta, Leslie Ciarleglio, and Amy Jarzebowicz for their perceptive reviews and suggestions. Patrick Clark provided graphic design. Skylar Sherwood, Debbie Olson, Leigh Elston, and Laura Burdell assisted with research, manuscript review, and moral support. The members of the NSGC Pedigree Standardization Task Force, particularly Kathryn Steinhaus, Stefanie Uhrich, Corrine O'Sullivan, and Debra Lochner-Doyle, helped seed the ideas for this book. I am grateful to the following individuals who took time from their busy schedules to review portions of the manuscript and provide valuable insights: Shari Baldinger, Dr. Thomas Bird, Dr. Peter Byers, Dr. Julie Gralow, Dr. Hanlee Ji, Dr. Gail Jarvik, Dr. Marshall Horwitz, Dr. Louanne Hudgins, Dr. Robert Kalina, Dr. Arno Motulsky, Dr. Roberta Pagon, Janine Polifka, Dr. Michael Raff, Dr. Al La Spada, Dr. C. Ronald Scott, Dr. Virginia Sybert, Ellen Nemens, Hillary Lipe, Marilyn Ray, Kathleen Delp, Joan Burns, Kerry Silvey and Linda Clapham. I appreciate the opportunity to work as a genetic counselor in the stimulating environment of the University of Washington, surrounded by a primordial soup of researchers in human genetics. My editors, Ann Boyle and Kristin Cooke, and the professionals at John Wiley and Sons have been generous in their patience and support. I thank my grandmother, Marjorie Warvelle Harbaugh, for teaching me respect and awe for my ancestors. Bill Tougaw, my high school biology teacher, deserves a special thank-you for opening my eyes and mind to the worlds of science and genetic counseling. I express my love and gratitude to my incredibly supportive family, especially Marjorie Bennett and J. J. Olsen, my husband Scott MacDonald, and my children, Colin, Evan, and Maren, for tolerating an "absent" Mom while I completed my dream.

Finally, I want to thank the families I have worked with through the years—you impress me with the strength you have in dealing with the cards life has dealt. Without question genes are important, but they are not our destiny. As Thomas Murry writes, "Why not regard our genes as a list of the obstacles we are likely to encounter and perhaps as a somewhat better prediction of how long we will have to do what matters to us, to be with the people we love, and to accomplish the tasks we have set for ourselves? Our genes no more dictate what is significant about our lives than the covers and pages of a blank diary dictate the content of what is written within. Our genes might be regarded metaphorically as the physical but blank, volume in which we will create our diary. Some volumes have fewer pages in which to write, some more. Certain pages, often toward the back of the volume may be more difficult to write on. And some leaves may require great skill and effort to open at all. But the physical volume is not the content of the diary. The content we must write ourselves."*

Robin L. Bennett
Seattle, Washington

*From TH Murry (1997). Genetic exceptionalism and "future diaries": Is genetic information different from other medical information? In: MA Rothstein (ed) *Genetic Secrets: Protecting Privacy and Confidentiality in the Genetic Era.* New Haven, London: Yale University Press.

1

The Language
of the Pedigree

Pedigrees are a challenge. With their intricate patterns of geometric symbols, pedigrees are like biological crossword puzzles which dare the clever and creative geneticist to solve them for clues about inheritance, family dynamics, or the localization of a gene.
—Robert G. Resta (1995)

WHY TAKE THE TIME TO RECORD A GENETIC FAMILY HISTORY?

The field of human genetics is revolutionizing the practice of medicine. The cyberspace bible of human genetics—Victor McKusick's *Online Mendelian Inheritance in Man* (better known as OMIM*)—lists more than 10,000 hereditary conditions! Identification of genetic mutations through the International Human Genome Project makes genetic testing for most of these conditions a reality. Genetic susceptibility mutations are now being identified as part of the causal nexus for common complex medical conditions such as cancer, diabetes, heart disease, Alzheimer disease, and mental illness. Human genetics is no longer just a topic for obscure medical journals. Headlines heralding genetic advances are splashed across the fronts of newspapers and popular magazines. The gripping stories of people making heartwrenching decisions about genetic testing and diagnosis increase the Nielsen ratings of Oprah Winfrey-style talk shows. Patients now come to *you* wanting to know if they need to worry about a genetic disease in their pregnancies, in their children, or in relation to their own health care.

How can you as a clinician identify individuals at risk for genetic disorders? The first step is to take a genetic family history, recorded in the shorthand form of a pedigree. A pedigree, commonly referred to as a family tree, is a graphic represen-

---

*http://www.ncbi.nlm.nih.gov/omim/

tation of a medical-family history using symbols. A concise pedigree provides both critical medical data and biological relationship information at a glance. In many circumstances, the pedigree is just as important for providing medical services to the patient as any laboratory test. The pedigree is truly the symbolic language of clinical genetic services and of human genetic research.

Genetic diseases affect all organ systems. Therefore health professionals from all specialties need to learn how to "think genetic." You do not need to be a "clever and creative geneticist" to take a genetic family history. The purpose of this book is to provide you with practical screening tools to make assessments as to which of your clients might benefit from more extensive genetic evaluation and/or testing. The goal is to teach you not just the questions to ask in making this assessment, but the logic behind these questions. Health professionals working with clients in family practice, internal medicine, pediatrics, and obstetrics will find these screening tools particularly useful. A special focus of this book is genetic screening questions for clinical specialists by disease system (see Chapter 4), with a particular emphasis on identifying individuals with an inherited susceptibility to cancer (see Chapter 5, and the cancer family history screening questionnaire in Appendix A.3). Researchers in human genetics will find useful information on how to obtain family history information, as well as ethical issues to consider in family studies and the publication of pedigrees (see Chapter 10). For the benefit of professionals involved in adoption, Chapter 7 discusses the unique issues surrounding a genetic family history and adoption. A medical-family history questionnaire for a child being placed for adoption is included in Appendix A.4.

WHAT DO CRANES HAVE TO DO WITH ANYTHING?

The word "pedigree" comes from the French term *pie de grue* or "crane's foot." The term first appeared in the English language in the 15th century. It described the curved lines, resembling a bird's claw, that were used to connect an individual with his or her offspring (Resta, 1993). Such vestiges of a bird's talons are obvious in the example of a *sippschaftstafel* drawn by Ernst Rüdin shown in Figure 1.1. The sippschaftstafel was a form of depicting family ancestry used by German eugenicists in the early 20th century (Mazumdar, 1992; Resta, 1993).

A pedigree is of limited value if the symbols and abbreviations cannot be easily interpreted. Historically, many different pedigree styles have been used in the published medical literature and in patient medical records (Bennett et al., 1993; Resta, 1993; Steinhaus et al., 1995). In fact, genetics professionals probably use as many "pedigree dialects" as there are dialects in the human language! As Francis Galton (an early geneticist and cousin to Charles Darwin) observed, "There are many methods of drawing pedigrees and describing kinship, but for my own purposes I still prefer those that I designed myself"(Galton, 1889). By using uniform symbols, it is possible to reduce the chances for incorrect interpretation of patient, family, medical, and genetic information. Through a peer-reviewed process, the Pedigree Standardization Task Force (PSTF) of the National Society of Genetic

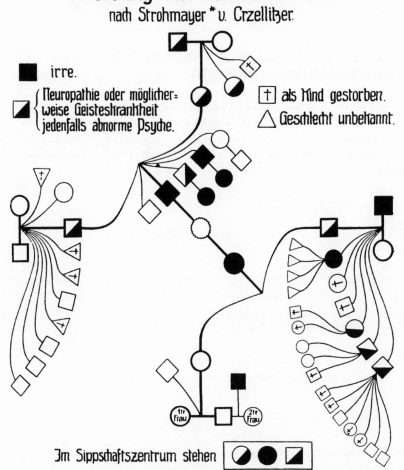

Figure 1.1   *A sippschaftstafel drawn by German eugenicist Ernst Rüdin in 1910. Note the proband (circle with irregular edge) is placed in the center of the pedigree and the maternal and paternal lineages radiate from curved lines drawn to the proband. Here the proband is shown being crushed by the weight of her dysgenic ancestry (from Mazumdar, 1992; and Resta, 1993). Reprinted with permission.*

Counselors (NSGC) developed standardized nomenclature for symbolizing pedigrees (Bennett et al., 1995). All pedigree symbols in this book conform to these standards.

THE PEDIGREE IS A COST-EFFECTIVE TOOL FOR GENETIC DIAGNOSIS AND RISK ASSESSMENT

"But who has time to take a family pedigree?" is a common lament from the busy practitioner. Most clinicians record some information about a patient's family illnesses in textual form. This can be just as time consuming as recording a pedigree, and the text may be much less concise, and much less specific, than a pedigree. For example, take a look at this excerpt from a medical record:

Linda's grandmother and two aunts died of breast cancer.

Did the cancer occur in Linda's maternal or paternal grandmother? Are the aunts the sisters of Linda's mother or Linda's father? The exact relationship of these affected relatives to Linda, their ages at death, and if the breast cancer was unilateral or bilateral can make a critical difference in your clinical assessment of Linda's risk for developing breast cancer. Instead, using the associative icons of a pedigree, the relevant family and medical information can be recorded quickly and precisely, in an easily interpretable format. A family pedigree is a tool for:

- Making a medical diagnosis
- Deciding on testing strategies
- Establishing the pattern of inheritance
- Identifying at-risk family members
- Calculating risks
- Determining reproductive options
- Distinguishing genetic from other risk factors
- Making decisions on medical management and surveillance
- Developing patient rapport
- Educating the patient
- Exploring the patient's understanding

Notation of a genetic family history is likely to become an essential component of a patient's medical record. The ability to elicit a comprehensive medical-family history, including drawing a family pedigree, is stated as a fundamental skill in providing familial cancer risk assessment by the American Society of Clinical Oncologists (ASCO, 1997). The American College of Obstetrics and Gynecology issued a similar statement on the importance of the genetic family history in obstetrical evaluations (ACOG, 1987). Dr. Peter Schwartz, Vice Chair of Obstetrics and Gynecology at Yale University School of Medicine, states that for early screening and detection of gynecologic malignancies, "Family history is crucial, and it's not a superficial history. You have to go into depth" (ACOG, 1998). Taking a directed genetic history is a primary step in the evaluation of most disorders. Dr. Barton Childs of Johns Hopkins University (1982) predicts that "to fail to take a good family history is bad medicine and someday will be criminal negligence."

Using a pedigree to symbolize a patient's medical and genetic history is no more time consuming than dictating a detailed summary for the medical chart. A pedigree is a way to compress pages and pages of medical information onto an $8\frac{1}{2}'' \times 11''$ piece of paper. I always keep the patient's pedigree in the front of his or her medical file. This saves me time at subsequent visits because most of the critical information I need is readily accessible and succinctly summarized on one page. The pedigree gives me an immediate image of the family's health and sociological structure without wading through stacks of medical records. Once a pedigree is obtained, the patient's family history can be easily updated on return visits.

The Pedigree as a Diagnostic Tool

Reviewing a family pedigree can aid the clinician in diagnosis. For example, in making a diagnosis of a familial cancer syndrome it is imperative to know the cluster of types of cancers; the ages of the individuals diagnosed with cancer; and how closely the individuals with cancer are related to each other (i.e., first- as compared to second-degree relatives). The family history will even influence the kind of genetic diagnostic tests that are ordered.

Take, for example, the family history of Susan, a 30-year-old computer technologist, and a mother of three. She is interested in information about how she can be screened for renal cell cancer because her father, Sam, was recently diagnosed with clear-cell renal carcinoma. If Susan has any family members with brain or spinal tumors (hemangioblastomas), renal cysts or cancer, adrenal tumors (pheochromocytomas), or retinal angiomas, a diagnosis of von Hippel–Lindau syndrome should be considered.

Von Hippel–Lindau syndrome (VHL) is an autosomal dominant condition with 80–90% penetrance and variable expressivity. Direct molecular genetic testing is available for VHL. With current molecular technology, about 80% of the mutations are identified (Huson and Rosser, 1997). Therefore, a negative molecular study does not rule out the diagnosis of VHL. A diagnosis of VHL in Sam will have very different implications for screening Susan, her children, and extended family, than does a diagnosis of an isolated clear-cell renal carcinoma. Isolated clear-cell renal carcinoma is not known to "run in families"—if Susan does not have additional family members with renal cell or other cancers, screening for any type of cancer in Susan will likely be the same as for any other woman her age (Linehan and Klausner, 1998). Susan's pedigree is depicted in Figure 1.2.

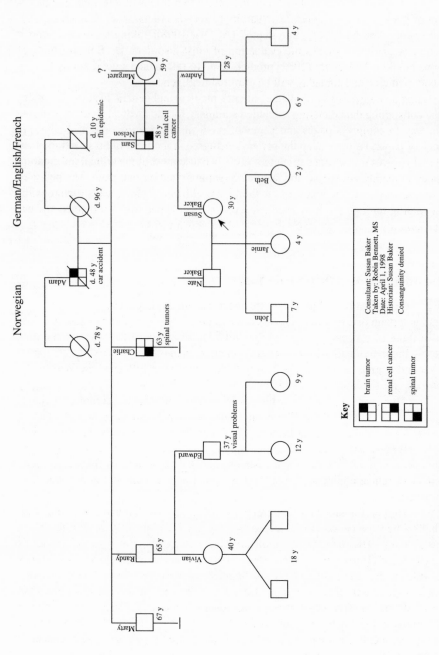

Figure 1.2 A hypothetical pedigree representative of a family with von Hippel–Lindau syndrome.

Using the Pedigree to Decide on Testing Strategies and for Evaluating At-risk Family Members

Susan's pedigree is suggestive of VHL. The most cost-effective approach to genetic testing is to obtain a blood sample from Sam to look for mutations in the VHL gene. Because VHL is inherited in an autosomal dominant pattern, an affected individual has a 50:50 chance to pass the mutation on to each son or daughter (see Chapter 2 for a review of patterns of inheritance). If a mutation is identified in Sam, then accurate mutation analysis is available for Susan, her siblings, and other family members. The pedigree helps you determine who else in the family should be tested.

Using the Pedigree to Establish the Pattern of Inheritance and to Calculate Risks

John was born with a profound hearing impairment. He and his fiancée are planning a family, and they want to know if they have a high probability of having children who will also have severe congenital hearing impairment. This question is impossible to answer without obtaining a family history. Congenital deafness can have an autosomal recessive, autosomal dominant, X-linked, or mitochondrial inheritance pattern, or have a maternal teratogenic etiology (see Chapter 4, Section 4.3). How to use a pedigree to identify patterns of inheritance is detailed in Chapter 2. Once an inheritance pattern is identified or suspected, John and his fiancée can be given appropriate genetic counseling.

A Pedigree Can Help Distinguish Genetic from Other Risk Factors

A pedigree can be just as useful in determining that a condition is *not* genetic as in establishing that a condition is inherited in a family. This is particularly true for common complex health conditions such as mental illness, heart disease, and cancer. For example, Jean is a 42-year-old premenopausal woman with unilateral breast cancer. Her mother is healthy at age 65 years, but Jean's maternal grandmother, Pamela, died of breast cancer at age 63. This limited family history may raise your initial suspicion for a familial breast cancer. Yet when you take an extended family history, you find that Jean's mother has three healthy sisters between the ages of 68 and 72 years. You also find that Pamela had two sisters who were cancer free in their mid-70s when they died of heart disease. This "negative" family history is just as important as the "positive" family history of cancer in risk assessment and determining cancer screening protocols.

A Pedigree Can Help Identify Medical Screening Needs for Healthy Individuals

A brief family history can identify genetic and medical screening needs for an otherwise healthy person. For example, carrier testing for Tay–Sachs disease can be offered to a healthy couple of Jewish ancestry who are interested in planning a pregnancy. (Tay-Sachs disease is an autosomal recessive neurodegenerative disease leading to death usually by the age of 5 years. Approximately 1 in 30 Ashkenazi Jews carries this mutation as compared to 1 in 300 individuals of non-Ashkenazi heritage.) Serum cholesterol screening can be considered for someone with a strong family history of coronary artery disease. For a person with a significant family history of colon cancer, colonoscopy should be offered at a younger age than usual (Burke et al., 1997b). A young woman with a strong family history of breast cancer should have screening mammography (or possibly breast ultrasounds) at an earlier age than is usually recommended (Burke et al., 1997a).

TAKING A FAMILY HISTORY IS A WAY TO ESTABLISH CLIENT RAPPORT AND FACILITATE PATIENT DECISION-MAKING

Your patients are more likely to comply with your medical advice if they trust you and have a relationship with you. The process of taking a medical-family history provides an excellent opportunity to establish rapport with a client. A clear picture of family dynamics and the patient's life experiences usually unfolds while taking a patient's medical-family history. These family relationships and life experiences will have an impact on a patient's decisions about medical care and genetic testing. Compare Amanda, a healthy 37-year-old pregnant woman who has experienced 10 years of infertility, with Beth, who is also 37 years old but has two healthy children. Both women have the same age-related risk to have a child with a chromosome anomaly, yet each woman may make different choices about genetic testing during her pregnancy. Or consider two 45-year-old women who each has a mother who died of breast cancer at age 38 years. Their genetic risk assessments (drawn from factual empiric risk tables) are the same, but the emotional feelings each woman has about medical screening and genetic testing are likely to differ based on each woman's individual experience with her mother's illness.

The symbols of a pedigree represent more than the geometric pieces of a biological crossword puzzle, as described by Robert Resta (1993) in the introductory quote to this chapter. I view a pedigree like a quilt, stitching together the intimate and colorful scraps of medical and family information from a person's life (Fig. 1.3). Familiar pedigree patterns are the clinician's matrix for providing pedigree risk assessment, as well as clinical and diagnostic recommendations. Yet just as the quilter takes artistic liberty with tried-and-true patterns to make each quilt a unique work of art, each pedigree has a unique human story behind it. It is from the interwoven fabric of a patient's family, cultural, and life experiences that the patient pieces together his or her decision-making framework.

A PEDIGREE CAN BE USED FOR PATIENT MEDICAL EDUCATION

"A picture is worth a thousand words," or so the popular saying goes. Reviewing the pedigree with a patient is a vital visual tool in patient education (Table 1.1). Let us

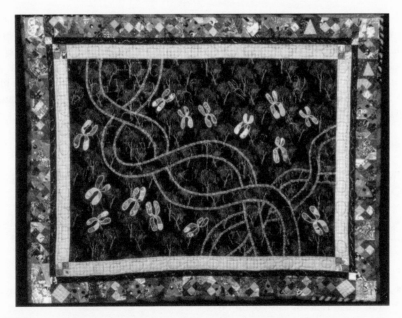

Figure 1.3   The Family Tree, *designed and stitched in 1997 by Josephine B. Rice of Gambier, Ohio in celebration of her grandson, Brian Alan Forthofer. Brian lived one day before dying from complications of trisomy 13 on March 7, 1997. Photographed by Ted Rice.*

return to Susan's family in Figure 1.2. Susan's pedigree can be used to explain autosomal dominant inheritance: there are people affected in more than one generation; both men and women are affected; and there is male-to-male transmission of the disease. To establish the diagnosis of VHL, you may want to obtain medical records on the people you suspect are affected in the family (such as Susan's father, her Uncle Charlie, and her paternal grandfather). By reviewing the pedigree with Susan, it is easy visually to show Susan family members which she needs to obtain medical records from, and why. The pedigree clearly defines who is at risk to develop VHL in Susan's family. You can discuss with Susan a plan for contacting extended family members. Strategies for helping a patient obtain medical records are presented in Chapter 6.

TABLE 1.1   The Pedigree As a Valuable Tool in Patient Education

The clinician can use a pedigree to:
- Review with the patient the need for obtaining medical documentation on affected family members
- Help the patient recognize the inheritance pattern of the disorder
- Provide a visual reminder of who in the family is at risk for the condition
- Demonstrate variability of disease expression (such as ages of onset)
- Assist the patient in exploring his or her understanding of the condition
- Clarify patient misconceptions

Reviewing a pedigree is an excellent tool for showing the variability of the disease expression in a family. In Susan's family it is obvious that some people with VHL have lived to an old age with few problems, whereas others are more severely affected. Susan's family history also nicely illustrates the various tumors that can occur together or in isolation. Seeing this visual representation of her family may help motivate Susan to follow your medical screening recommendations because, with a glance, she is reminded of the impact that VHL has had on her extended family.

USING A PEDIGREE TO EXPLORE A PATIENT'S UNDERSTANDING AND TO CLARIFY MISCONCEPTIONS

Reviewing the pedigree with Susan is an excellent way to explore Susan's feelings about being at risk for VHL, as well as her understanding of the disease:

- What about genetic testing and medical screening for Susan's children?
- How will Susan feel if she finds she is affected with VHL and now her children are at risk for this condition?
- If Susan has VHL, what type of support does she have from her extended family to deal with her chronic illness?
- How will Susan feel if she is unaffected with VHL yet her sister is affected, or vice versa?

Almost invariably, a person seeking information about a genetic disease or genetic testing has already reached some of his or her own conclusions about the inheritance of their "family's curse." In fact, considerable family lore may center on complicated theories about the inheritance of the disease in question. For example, Susan might think that she is not at risk for VHL in her family because mostly men are affected. You can point out to Susan that her father did not have any sisters. Or Susan may falsely believe that the eldest sibling is spared from disease. A pedigree is a wonderful way to clarify patient misconceptions. Table 1.2 lists many of the common misconceptions patients have about the inheritance of a condition in their family.

THE CONTINUING EVOLUTION OF THE PEDIGREE IN THE AGE OF GENOMIC MEDICINE

Thanks to the International Human Genome Project, the genes of the human genome are likely to be located and sequenced by the year 2003. The ability to practice genomic medicine, by potentially viewing the molecular status of each patient's individual genome, has an impact on all medical disciplines. Yet it is absurd to think

TABLE 1.2   Common Patient Misconceptions about Inheritance

∅ If no one else in the family is affected, the condition is not inherited.

∅ If several people in the family have the same condition, it must be inherited.

∅ All birth defects are inherited.

∅ The parents (particularly the mother) must have done something before conception or during the pregnancy to "cause" the condition in their fetus or child.

∅ With a 25% recurrence risk, after one affected child, the next three will be unaffected.

∅ With a 50% recurrence risk, every other child is affected.

∅ Birth order influences disease status (for example, only the eldest or youngest child can be affected).

∅ If the affected individuals in the family are all women, or all men, the condition must be sex-linked.

∅ A person will inherit the genetic condition because he or she "looks" or "acts" like the affected relative(s). Or the opposite—a person will not inherit a condition because he or she bears no resemblance to the affected relative(s).

∅ For a condition with sex-influenced expression (such as breast cancer), individuals of the opposite sex cannot transmit the condition (for example, a male cannot pass on a gene alteration for breast cancer).

Source: Revised from Connor and Ferguson-Smith, 1997.

that a complete genomic reference map will then lead us to the understanding of all that is human or that we are the direct and inevitable consequence of our genome. The genetic family history will continue to play an essential role in the medicine of the 21st century. As Dr. Reed Pyeritz (1997), President of the American College of Medical Genetics, succinctly summarizes:

> The importance of the family history will only be enhanced in the future. Even when an individual's genome can be displayed on a personal microchip, interpreting that information will depend in large part, on the biological and environmental contexts in which the genome is expressed, and the family milieu is as good a guide as any. Physicians can help define those contexts through careful family and social histories. How those histories can be obtained and interpreted, when the average time for patient interaction with a physician continues to diminish, are crucial areas for research.

Variation is the hallmark of humans—even within well-established diseases with known patterns of inheritance, there is remarkable disease variability. Pedigree assessment will continue to play a critical role in our understanding of gene expression. A patient who has a genetic disorder, or one who carries a genetic susceptibility mutation, cannot be viewed in isolation from the background of his or her family history. How is it that five relatives with the same gene mutation can all have different ages of onset and varying manifestations of the same genetic disorder? The patient and his or her genotype must be examined in the context of his or her genetic and environmental exposures. The clues from buried ancestors can reach out to the present to provide solutions for the future.

REFERENCES

American College of Obstetricians and Gynecologists (1987). Antenatal diagnosis of genetic disorders (ACOG Technical Bulletin 108). Washington DC: ACOG.

American College of Obstetricians and Gynecologists (1998), Stone ML (ed). Screening and early detection of gynecologic malignancies (ACOG Update Vol 23). Washington DC: ACOG.

American Society of Clinical Oncologists (1997). Resource document for curriculum development in cancer genetics education. J Clin Oncol 15:2157–2169.

Bennett RL, Steinhaus KA, Uhrich SB, O'Sullivan C (1993). The need for developing standardized family pedigree nomenclature. J Genet Couns 2:261–273.

Bennett RL, Steinhaus KA, Uhrich SB, et al. (1995). Recommendations for standardized human pedigree nomenclature. Am J Hum Genet 56(3):745–752.

Burke W, Daly M, Garber J, et al. (1997a). Recommendations for follow-up care of individuals with an inherited predisposition to cancer II. BRCA1 and BRCA2. JAMA 227:997–1003.

Burke W, Petersen G, Lynch P, et al. (1997b) Recommendations for follow-up care of individuals with an inherited predisposition to cancer I. Hereditary nonpolyposis colon cancer. JAMA 277(11):915–919.

Childs B (1982). Genetics in the medical curriculum. Am J Med Genet 13:319–324.

Connor M, Ferguson-Smith M (1997). *Essential Medical Genetics*, 5th ed. Oxford: Blackwell Science.

Galton F (1889). *Natural Inheritance*. London: MacMillan.

Huson SM, Rosser, EM (1997). The phakomatoses. In Rimoin DL, Connor JM, Pyeritz RE (eds), *Emery and Rimoin's Principles and Practice of Medical Genetics*, 3rd ed. New York: Churchill Livingstone, pp. 2269–2302.

Linehan WM, Klausner RD (1998). Renal carcinoma. In Vogelstein B, Kinzler KW (eds), *The Genetic Basis of Human Cancer*. New York: McGraw Hill, pp. 455–473.

Mazumdar PMH (1992). *Eugenics, Human Genetics and Human Failings*. London, New York: Routledge.

Online Mendelian Inheritance in Man, OMIM (TM). Center for Medical Genetics, Johns Hopkins University (Baltimore, MD) and National Center for Biotechnology Information, National Library of Medicine (Bethesda, MD), 1997. Accessed June 19, 1998. World Wide Web URL: http://www.ncbi.nlm.nih.gov/omim/

Pyeritz RE (1997). Family history and genetic risk factors. Forward to the future. JAMA 278 (15):1284–1285.

Resta RG (1993). The crane's foot: The rise of the pedigree in human genetics. J Genet Couns 2(4):235–260.

Resta RG (1995). Whispered hints. Am J Med Genet 59:131–133.

Steinhaus KA, Bennett RL, Uhrich SB, et al. (1995). Inconsistencies in pedigree nomenclature in human genetics publications: a need for standardization. Am J Med Genet 56(5):291–295.

2

Practical Inheritance

*No genetic factor works in a void, but in an environment
which may help or hinder its expression.*
—*Eliot Slater (1936)*

THE MYTH OF MENDEL

In some far-off recess of each human mind hides the Mendelian rules of inheritance
that we learned in our early school education. Like many ideas of the 1860s, the
principles of Gregor Mendel do not reflect the changing times. Should we be sur-
prised that inheritance patterns in humans are more complex than in garden peas, or
that an Augustinian monk is an unlikely resource on matters of human reproduction?

Mendel's laws work under the simple assumptions that genetic factors are transmitted from each parent as discrete units that are inherited independently from one
another and passed (unaltered) from one generation to the next. Thus begins the
myth of Mendel. We now know that genes do not function in isolation, but interact
with each other and the environment (for example, modifying genes and regulating
elements of genes). Genes that are in close proximity to each other may be inherited
as a unit rather than independently (such as in *contiguous gene syndromes*). Some
genes are indeed altered from one generation to the next, as is evidenced by *dynamic mutations* (seen in *trinculeotide repeat disorders*), new mutations, and *parental
imprinting*. Mendelian principles really become obsolete when applied to *mitochondrial inheritance* because in this instance there is no paternal genetic contribution!

Despite these caveats, it is still useful to divide hereditary conditions into three
classic inheritance patterns: single gene (classic Mendelian), multifactorial or polygenic, and chromosomal. Single gene disorders are classified by whether they are
dominant or recessive and by their locations on the chromosomes. Genes for autosomal disorders are on one of the 22 pairs of non-sex chromosomes (*autosomes*).
Genes for *sex-linked* disorders are on the X or Y chromosomes. *Sporadic* inheri-

tance usually refers to the one-time occurrence of a condition. In this instance, unaffected siblings usually do not have affected children but the parents may have a risk of recurrence due to factors such as *gonadal mosaicism* and parental imprinting.

Do not panic if you think mosaicism applies only to tile floors in Mexico, imprinting is the latest craze in rubber stamps, or dynamic mutations are the action-figure stars of a Saturday morning cartoon. Clues for identifying the standard (and not-so-standard) patterns of inheritance are reviewed in Table 2.1. Included in this chapter are representative pedigrees for the primary inheritance patterns as well as tables with a sampling of common genetic conditions and their estimated incidences (See Tables 2.2–2.4).

A BRIEF GENETICS PRIMER

Here are some general points to remember from the day that you may have been drifting off in your genetics lecture:

Humans carry an estimated 60,000–100,000 expressed genes. Genes are the basic chemical units of heredity. They are packaged in rows (like beads on a string) on rodlike structures called chromosomes in the cell nucleus. Each gene has a specific place or *locus* on the chromosome. Every person inherits one copy of a gene from his (or her) mother and one from the father. Alternative copies of the same gene are called *alleles*. The *genotype* is an individual's genetic constitution. The *phenotype* is the observed physical expression (physical, biochemical, and physiological) of an individual's genotype.

Humans have 23 pairs of chromosomes in each cell of the body except the egg and sperm, which have only one copy of each chromosome. There are 22 pairs of non-sex chromosomes called autosomes. The 23rd pair of chromosomes, the sex chromosomes, are called X and Y. Females have two X chromosomes. Males have an X and a Y chromosome. The centromeres are the sites of attachment of the spindle fibers during cell division. A centromere divides a chromosome into a short (upper) arm called the "p" arm and a long (lower) arm called the "q" arm.

A gene begins as a molecule of DNA (deoxyribonucleic acid). There are four "letters" (called nitrogenous bases) in the DNA alphabet: A (adenine), C (cytosine), G (guanine), and T (thymine). Nucleotides are composed of a nitrogenous base, a sugar molecule, and a phosphate molecule. The nitrogenous bases pair together—A with T, and G with C—like rungs on a ladder, with the sugar and phosphates serving as the backbone. The DNA ladder is shaped in a twisted helix. The DNA helix unzips and free nucleotides join the single-stranded DNA to form a matching ribonucleic acid molecule called mRNA in a process called transcription. The initial mRNA "sense" strand matches the complementary "anti-sense" DNA template with the exception that thymine (T) is replaced by uracil (U).

There are coding regions of DNA (*exons*) and noncoding regions of DNA (*introns*). Most DNA is noncoding. The DNA molecule also has regulatory regions, such as those for "starting" and "stopping" transcription and translation, and specialized sequences related to tissue-specific expression. The initial mRNA (or pri-

TABLE 2.1 Pedigree Clues for Distinguishing the Primary Patterns of Human Inheritance

Inheritance Pattern	Pedigree Clues
Autosomal dominant	Male-to-male transmission Condition seen in multiple successive generations Males and females affected Often see variability in severity of clinical disease expression Affected individuals may have late age of clinical onset Homozygotes may be more severely affected than heterozygotes Homozygous state may be lethal
Autosomal recessive	Affected individuals usually just in one generation Sometimes see parental consanguinity Males and females affected May be mistaken for sporadic occurrence if small family size Symptoms often seen in newborn, infancy, or early childhood Disease may be more common in certain ethnic groups Often inborn errors of metabolism
X-linked dominant	Often lethal in males, so see a paucity of males in pedigree May see multiple miscarriages (because of lethality in males) Females usually express condition, but have milder symptoms No male-to-male transmission
X-linked recessive	Males affected Females may be affected, but usually much milder than males May be "missed" if paucity of females in family No male-to-male transmission

Chromosomal	Suspect in a person with two or more major birth defects,
	   three or more minor birth defects,
	   or one major and two minor birth defects
	A fetus with a major structural anomaly
	Unexplained mental retardation (static) especially in a person with dysmorphic features
	Unexplained psychomotor retardation
	Ambiguous genitalia
	Lymphedema or cystic hygroma in a newborn
	Multiple pregnancy losses
	Family history of mental retardation and individuals with multiple congenital anomalies
	Unexplained infertility

Contiguous gene	Mental retardation with other recognized genetic or medical conditions Recognized single gene condition with uncharacteristic dysmorphic features Family history usually unremarkable
Mitochondrial	Father does not transmit condition to children; only mother does Highly variable clinical expressivity Often central nervous system disorders Males and females affected, often in multiple generations May be degenerative
Multifactorial	Males and females affected No clear pattern Skips generations Few affected family members

mary transcript) is modified before diffusing to the cytoplasm so that the final mRNA is composed only of exons (the introns are spliced out during mRNA processing).

The mRNA molecule diffuses to the cytoplasm where it is translated into a polypeptide chain by the ribosomes. Each mRNA codon is recognized by a matching complementary tRNA anticodon that is attached to a corresponding amino acid. For example, the DNA sequence "GCT" is transcribed into the mRNA sequence "CGU." The mRNA sequence "CGU" is read on the ribosomes by the tRNA anticodon "GCA," which attaches the amino acid arginine to the growing polypeptide chain. The sequence of the 20 amino acids determines the form and function of the resulting protein (e.g., structural protein, enzyme, carrier molecule, receptor molecule, hormone). Proteins usually undergo further modification after ribosomal translation (e.g., phosphorylation, proteolytic cleavage, glycosylation).

Each cell contains hundreds of mitochondria in the cytoplasm. Mitochondria are the "powerhouses" of the cells and are essential for energy metabolism. Each mitochondrion has about 10 single copies of small, circular chromosomes. These chromosomes consist of double-stranded helices of DNA (mtDNA). Human mtDNA has only exons, and both strands of DNA are transcribed and translated.

All mitochondria are maternally inherited. The mitochondria in each cell are derived at the time of fertilization from the mitochondria in the cytoplasm of the ovum. Sperm do not contribute mitochondria or mtDNA at fertilization.

Single gene disorders arise as a result of a mutation in one or both alleles of a gene located in an autosome, a sex chromosome, or a mitochondrial gene. A person who has identical alleles for a gene is *homozygous*, and an individual in whom the alleles are not identical is *heterozygous*. Because the X and Y chromosomes do not have homologous (matching) genes, males are said to be *hemizygous* for genes on the X and Y chromosomes.

Single gene disorders generally refer to conditions inherited in patterns that follow the rules originally described by Gregor Mendel. These traditional Mendelian patterns are autosomal dominant (AD), autosomal recessive (AR), X-linked recessive (XLR), X-linked dominant (XLD), and Y-linked. *Chromosomal disorders* are present if there is a visible alteration in the number or structure of the chromosomes. *Multifactorial inheritance* refers to the complex interplay of genetic and environmental factors. *Polygenic inheritance* describes the effects of two or more genes, usually in combination with environmental factors, which are involved in the expression of a trait. As we recognize more readily the contributions of genes interacting with the environment and with each other, the boundary between single gene disorders and multifactorial disorders continues to blur.

CONFOUNDING FACTORS IN RECOGNIZING PATTERNS OF INHERITANCE

Failure to obtain complete medical-family history information from a patient may compromise the clinician's ability to recognize an inheritance pattern. With few exceptions, the pedigree should extend at least three generations to include the patient's grandparents, parents, siblings, half siblings, nieces and nephews, children, grandchildren, and aunts and uncles (see Chapter 3). Remember to record the ages, sex, and health information of both affected and unaffected relatives. *Information on unaffected relatives is just as important as information on affected relatives.* For example, if you take a history of a 50-year-old woman diagnosed with unilateral breast cancer at age 42 years, and she has four sisters cancer-free in their 60s, you are more likely to consider this cancer a sporadic occurrence than to suspect an autosomal dominant inheritance pattern.

A person with only mild clinical symptoms may be missed as being affected in a pedigree. *Variable expressivity* means that the clinical severity of a disorder differs from one individual to another. For example, two siblings with cystic fibrosis (an autosomal recessive condition characterized by pancreatic insufficiency and progressive accumulation of mucus in the lungs) may each have very different manifestations of the disease. It is not uncommon for the seemingly healthy sibling of a child with cystic fibrosis to be diagnosed serendipitously through molecular genetic testing rather than by clinical symptoms.

Recognizing that individuals within a family have the same genetic syndrome is also confounded by *clinical* or *genetic heterogeneity*. This means that individuals with similar phenotypes can have entirely different genetic causes. For example, ovarian cancer is usually not inherited, but of the 3–13% that is familial, mutations in multiple cancer susceptibility genes associated with ovarian cancer have been identified: BRCA1, BRCA2, hereditary non-polyposis colon cancer (HNPCC), Peutz–Jeghers syndrome, and basal cell nevus syndrome (DePasquale et al., 1998; Houlston et al., 1992).

The expression of a syndrome may be influenced by the sex of an individual even when the gene is located on a non-sex chromosome. This is called *sex-influenced* or *sex-limited gene expression*. For example, it may be difficult to recognize families with an inherited breast cancer susceptibility if most of the people in the family are men because men rarely develop breast cancer. The breast cancer mutation can be inherited through healthy men in a family.

The practical 6-year-old who states, "One of the people has freckles and so he finds someone else who has freckles too," unknowingly describes the definition of *assortative mating*. Humans do not choose a mating partner randomly. We tend to have children with people from similar cultural and ethnic backgrounds. It is not unusual for people with comparable medical challenges to have children together. For example, two people with the same condition, such as deafness or short stature, may have children together. Because there are multiple etiologies for either of these conditions, it may be difficult to determine an inheritance pattern and provide appropriate genetic counseling.

To heir is human. Nonpaternity is probably the primary explanation for confusion in pedigree interpretation. The rate of nonpaternity in the United States is estimated to be as high as 10%. Misattribution of fatherhood crosses all racial and socioeconomic groups. In some circumstances it may be important for the clinician to verify paternity with DNA testing.

Small family size is an obvious problem in recognizing patterns of inheritance. In a family where both healthy parents are only children, and their affected child has no siblings, it may be impossible to distinguish a pattern of inheritance.

Other potential explanations for a seemingly "negative" family history are listed in Table 3.4.

RECOGNIZING PATTERNS OF INHERITANCE

Dominant and Recessive Inheritance Patterns: A Shifting Paradigm

Historically, *dominant inheritance* is the term used when the heterozygote and homozygote are clinically indistinguishable. In other words, only one copy of the gene mutation or alteration is needed for clinical (*phenotypic*) features. Recessive inheritance traditionally describes individuals who are clinically affected when they have a "double dose" (homozygosity) of a gene alteration. The ability to examine gene action at the biochemical and molecular levels demonstrates that gene expression is not strictly dominant or recessive; each allele can have distinct phenotypic expression. Thus there can be phenotypic expression of both alleles in the heterozygous state. Many human geneticists describe this as *co-dominant inheritance, semi-dominant inheritance*, or *intermediate expression* (Strachan and Read, 1996; Vogel and Motulsky, 1996). Although the expression of any "trait" or "character" requires the expression of multiple genes and environmental factors, if a particular genotype is sufficient for the trait to be expressed, the trait is considered to be inherited in a Mendelian pattern.

Autosomal Dominant Inheritance

Conditions inherited in an autosomal dominant (AD) pattern account for approximately half of all single gene disorders. In AD inheritance (Fig. 2.1) an affected individual has a 50:50 chance to pass the gene mutation to each son or daughter. Multiple people of both sexes are usually affected in more than one generation. A key feature that identifies AD inheritance is transmission of the trait from father to son (*male-to-male transmission*). Many AD conditions have *variable expression*. Because a parent and other extended relatives may have only minor features of the condition, *it is crucial to examine both parents for subtle symptoms of the disease in question*.

The recognition of an AD pattern can be complicated by the *penetrance* of the trait. Penetrance refers to the percentage likelihood that an individual who has inherited a gene mutation will actually show the disease manifestations in his or her lifetime. Some conditions are fully penetrant at birth, meaning the condition is either evident or not at birth. For example, an AD cleft lip and palate syndrome may have a penetrance of 40%. Thus an unaffected person in such a family would have a high probability to carry a "hidden" mutation that could be passed to a child. Other conditions are penetrant by a certain age. For example, familial adenomatous poly-

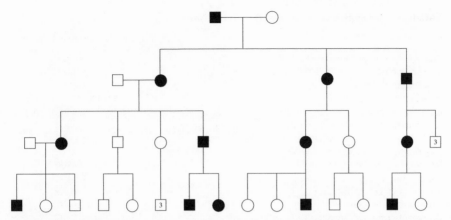

Figure 2.1 *Representative pedigree of autosomal dominant (AD) inheritance. Note male-to-male disease transmission and affected individuals of both sexes in successive generations.*

posis (FAP) is an AD colon cancer syndrome that is 100% penetrant by the age of 40 years. Thus anyone with an FAP gene mutation should have hundreds of colonic polyps by age 40 years, but a 5-year-old child with the gene mutation may have no observable manifestations.

If two people with the same AD condition have children together, there is a 75% chance with each pregnancy that they will have an affected son or daughter. There is a 25% chance that they will have a child who has a "double dose" of the mutation (homozygosity). In some instances, the child with a homozygous mutation may be very severely affected by the condition. For other conditions, such as achondroplasia (an AD disproportionate short stature syndrome), the homozygous state is lethal.

Many AD conditions, such as neurofibromatosis, Marfan syndrome, and retinoblastoma, have a frequent new mutation rate. Thus an individual can be the first person in the family with the condition. This means that the mutation occurred in the egg or sperm from which the person was conceived. The person who has the condition has a 50:50 chance to pass the condition on to each of his or her children, but the person's brothers and sisters are usually not at risk for the condition. The exception is if one of the parents is mosaic for the mutation in the testes or ovaries. This phenomenon of *gonadal mosaicism* is discussed in more detail near the end of this chapter, under the topic of mosaicism.

Table 2. 2 lists some conditions with AD inheritance.

Autosomal Recessive Inheritance

Parents who each carry an autosomal recessive (AR) gene mutation have a 25% chance, with each conception, to have an affected son or daughter. Many inborn errors of metabolism are inherited in an AR pattern. Consanguinity can be a clue to an

TABLE 2.2   Examples of Autosomal Dominant Conditions

Condition	Approximate Prevalence
Familial hypercholesterolemia	1/500
Adult polycystic kidney disease	1/1000
Von Willebrand disease	1/1000
Polydactyly (postaxial)	1/3000 (Caucasians)
Neurofibromatosis 1	1/3500
Oculo-auriculo-vertebral spectrum (hemifacial microsomia)	1/5600
Charcot–Marie–Tooth type I/hereditary motor sensory neuropathy (heterogeneous)	1/6600
Myotonic muscular dystrophy	1/7500
Familial adenomatous polyposis (FAP or APC)	1/8000
Tuberous sclerosis complex	1/10,000
Dominant blindness	1/10,000
Dominant congenital deafness	1/10,000
Achondroplasia	1/10,000–1/15,000
Marfan syndrome	1/16,000–1/25,000
Osteogenesis imperfecta (all types)	1/20,000
Huntington disease	1/20,000
Waardenburg syndrome	1/33,000–1/50,000
Van der Woude syndrome	1/35,000
Von Hippel–Lindau syndrome	1/36,000

Sources: Connor and Ferguson-Smith, 1997; Gorlin et al., 1990; Offit, 1998; Rimoin et al., 1997; Robinson and Linden, 1993; Scriver et al., 1995.

AR pattern because individuals who are closely related are more likely to have inherited the same AR gene mutation from a common ancestor. All humans are estimated to carry several "hidden" AR gene mutations (Fig. 2.2).

Some AR conditions are common in certain ethnic groups because individuals of the same background are more likely to have children together (see Chapter 3, Table 3.2). For example Tay–Sachs disease has a 1/30 carrier frequency in the Ashkenazi Jewish population (Jews from Eastern and Central Europe), versus a 1/300 carrier frequency in the non-Ashkenazi population. Cystic fibrosis has a frequency of 1/3300 in individuals of Northern European ancestry, 1/15,300 in individuals of African American ancestry (a carrier frequency of approximately 1/60–65), and about 1/50,000 in Native Africans (NIH Consensus, 1997).

The siblings of parents who are known carriers of an autosomal recessive trait have a one in two (50%) risk to be carriers. The unaffected siblings of individuals with AR conditions have a two in three (66%) chance to be carriers. The chance that these individuals will have affected children depends upon the chance that their partners carry the same AR gene mutation. This chance will be higher if the partner is a "blood relative" (e.g., a cousin), or if he or she is from a population group where the carrier frequency for the disease is high. For most rare AR conditions, the chance that healthy siblings will have children with the condition is low (in the range of 1% or less). Likewise, individuals with autosomal recessive conditions usually do not have children who are affected, although *all* their children are obligate carriers of the gene mutation. Depending on the carrier frequency of the gene al-

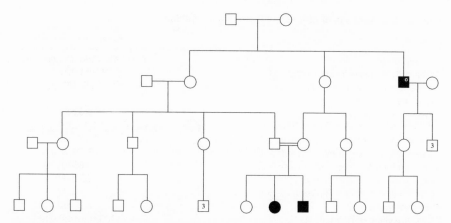

Figure 2.2 *Representative pedigree of autosomal recessive (AR) inheritance. Although consanguinity is a clue suggesting AR inheritance, most individuals with an AR condition are born to unrelated parents.*

teration, the risk that these children will be affected usually is in the range of 0.5–3%.

Table 2.3 lists some common conditions that are inherited in an AR pattern.

X-linked Inheritance

Women who carry an X-chromosome gene mutation have a 50:50 chance, with each pregnancy, to have an affected son. Also, there is a 50:50 chance with each pregnancy to have a daughter who carries the mutation. Usually daughters are unaffected. A pedigree where only males are affected, often in more than one generation, is a key to detecting a traditional *X-linked recessive* (XLR) inheritance pattern. The family history for an XLR disorder may show few affected family members, particularly if most of the family members are female (Fig. 2.3).

The concept of dominant and recessive inheritance blurs when applied to X-linked inheritance. Heterozygous women can be affected with an XLR condition, but usually they are more mildly affected than their male relatives are. The main explanation for this is *lyonization* or *X-inactivation*. Inactivation of one of the X-chromosomes occurs soon after fertilization when the embryo contains several hundred to several thousand cells. A single X chromosome remains active per cell. This inactivation is a random process. If the clones of these original cells carry the inactive X with the normally working gene, then the woman may have symptoms of the condition. For example, women who carry the X-linked recessive Duchenne muscular dystrophy (DMD) mutation may have subtle symptoms of DMD (such as large calves and high blood levels of the contractile muscle enzyme, creatine kinase). Affected boys, in contrast, will have highly elevated creatine kinase levels at birth and progressive muscle weakness, such that they usually require wheelchair assistance by the age of 10–12 years (Emery, 1997).

TABLE 2.3   Examples of Autosomal Recessive Conditions

Condition	Approximate Prevalence[a]
Hemochromatosis	1/300–1/500 (Caucasians)
Sickle cell anemia (African Americans)	1/400–1/600
β–thalassemia (Italian or Greek Americans)	1/800–1/2000
Cystic fibrosis	
Northern Europeans	1/3300
African Americans	1/15,000
Asian Americans	1/32,100
Nonsyndromic neurosensory deafness (DFNB1)	1/5000
Medium-chain-acyl-dehydrogenase (MCAD)	1/6000
Alpha-1 antitrypsin deficiency	1/4400–1/8000
Spinal muscular atrophy I (Werdnig–Hoffman)	1/10,000
Phenylketonuria (PKU)	1/12,000
21-Hydroxylase deficiency	1/8000–1/26,000
Albinism (all types)	1/20,000
Smith–Lemli–Opitz syndrome	1/20,000
Infantile polycystic kidney disease	1/20,800
Usher syndrome	1/23,000–1/33,000
Glutaric aciduria (Northern European)	1/30,000
Galactosemia	1/40,000
Homocystinuria	1/200,000
Tay–Sachs disease (non-Jewish)	1/300,000
Ashkenazi Jewish	1/3300

[a]The frequency of these diseases may vary widely among ethnic groups. Table 3.2 in Chapter 3 lists some autosomal recessive conditions that have a high frequency within certain population groups.
Sources: Clarke, 1996; Connor and Ferguson-Smith, 1997; NIH Consensus Statement, 1997; Offit, 1998; Rimoin et al., 1997; Scriver et al., 1995.

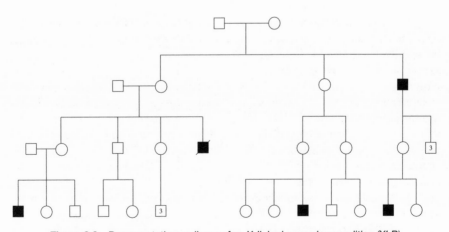

Figure 2.3   *Representative pedigree of an X-linked recessive condition (XLR).*

There are some X-linked conditions, particularly those involving enzyme defi-ciencies, in which it is common for heterozygous carriers to show mild symptoms (intermediate expression). For example, women who are carriers for nephrogenic diabetes insipidus (hereditary renal tubular insensitivity to antidiuretic hormone) often show symptoms of increased thirst for water, and dilute urine. The affected males, on the other hand, are treated with free access to water, diuretics, and a low-sodium diet to prevent repeated bouts of hypernatremia, potentially leading to fail-ure to thrive and mental retardation (Reeves and Andreoli, 1995). Ornithine tran-scarbamylase deficiency (OTCD, a urea cycle defect leading to hyperammonemia) is usually lethal in males in the first few years of life, even with strict protein re-striction and dietary arginine. The female carriers may have protein intolerance, but rarely require treatment.

X-linked dominant inheritance traditionally describes conditions where the het-erozygous female manifests disease symptoms, and the condition is usually lethal (in utero or in infancy) for the male *hemizygote*. In this instance, the pedigree clues include only females being affected, and multiple miscarriages (representing in utero death of a male fetus) (see Fig. 2.4). These conditions are rare. An example of such a condition is incontinentia pigmenti. Female infants with this condition have blisters that spontaneously resolve, leaving marbled brown or slate gray pigmenta-tion that fades into hypopigmented macules in an adult. Other features may include hypodontia (congenital absence of primary or secondary teeth), partial hair loss (alopecia), mental delay, and ocular problems. The condition is lethal in males (Sybert, 1997).

A family history of an X-linked condition in which the women express the con-dition is distinguishable from AD inheritance by the absence of male-to-male trans-

TABLE 2.4   Examples of X-linked Conditions.

Condition	Approximate Prevalence (Males)
Red–green color blindness (Europeans)	8/100
Fragile X syndrome	1/2000–1/2500
Duchenne muscular dystrophy	1/3000–1/5000
Hemophilia A (factor VIII)	1/2500–1/4000
Hemophilia B (Christmas disease, Factor IX)	1/4000–1/7000
Vitamin D resistant rickets (X-linked hypophosphatemia)	1/25,000
Fabry disease	1/40,000
Hunter syndrome (MPS II)	1/144,000
Orofacial digital syndrome I[a]	1/50,000
Ornithine transcarbamylase deficiency[a] (males usually die in first few years of life)	1/20,000–1/30,000
?Rett syndrome (lethal in males)	1/10,000 (females)
Nephrogenic diabetes insipidus[a]	1/30,000–1/50,000 (about 10% are autosomal recessive)
Incontinentia pigmenti[a] (lethal in males)	rare

[a]Disorders that are traditionally considered X-linked dominant.
Sources: Connor and Ferguson-Smith, 1997; Rimoin et al., 1997; Scriver et al., 1995.

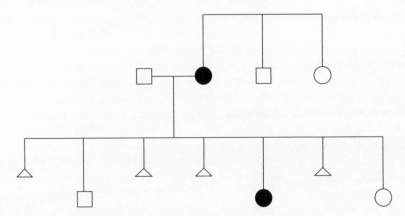

Figure 2.4 *Pedigree suggestive of an X-linked mutation that is lethal in males. Note the absence of affected males and the multiple pregnancy losses.*

mission (see Fig. 2.5). Male-to-male transmission can be mimicked in pedigrees where there is consanguinity (a union between relatives) because an affected father may have children with a female relative who is a carrier for the same condition; thus sons can inherit the gene alteration from the mother. Another feature that distinguishes an X-linked pedigree from autosomal dominant pedigrees is that in X-linked conditions the females are generally more mildly affected than the males, whereas in AD conditions, both men and women may have variable expression of the disease.

Because men pass the X chromosome only to their daughters, the daughters of a man with an X-linked condition are always carriers (and rarely affected), and their

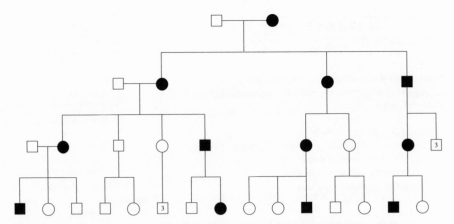

Figure 2.5 *Representative pedigree of X-linked dominant inheritance. Note that males and females are affected, and that males have affected daughters but no affected sons. Usually the females have less severe manifestations than their male relatives.*

sons are never affected. The carrier daughters each have a 50:50 risk to have an affected son. Thus the grandsons of these carrier males are at risk to be affected.

Similar to AD conditions, many X-linked conditions have a high new mutation rate. For those X-linked conditions causing severe physical impairment in which it is unusual for affected men to father children, the new mutation rates are often 20–30%. For example, if a woman has a son with Duchenne muscular dystrophy and there are no other affected family members, the chance that her affected son has a new mutation in the dystrophin gene is approximately 1/3.

Y-Inheritance (Holandric)

The Y chromosome is small. It contains only a short segment of functional genes that are largely responsible for determining maleness (autosomal genes are also associated with sex determination). A gene on the short arm of the chromosome called the SRY (sex-determining region of Y) mediates the male-determining effect of the Y chromosome. Genetic alterations in this segment can affect human sex differentiation, leading to such conditions as XY females and XX males. Alterations in the SRY gene and other gene loci on the Y chromosome may be responsible for hereditary infertility (Vogel and Motulsky, 1996; Okabe et al., 1998). Genetic causes of male infertility are reviewed in greater detail in Chapter 4, Section 4.16.

Multifactorial and Polygenic Disorders

Multifactorial conditions are believed to have both environmental and genetic components. Multiple genes may play a role in the expression of the condition (polygenic inheritance). Height and skin color are good examples of conditions in which multiple genes and the environment are involved in phenotypic expression. Many isolated birth defects such as pyeloric stenosis, clubfoot, scoliosis, and neural tube defects are believed to have a multifactorial etiology. Common illnesses in adults, such as diabetes, asthma, hypertension, epilepsy, and mental disorders are also thought to have multiple genetic and environmental factors at the root of their expression.

Pedigrees documenting conditions that have a multifactorial or polygenic etiology usually have no other, or few, affected family members (Fig. 2.6). Males and females may be affected. The risk of recurrence is based on empirical data tables derived from population studies. The more closely related a person is to the affected individual, the higher the chance of being affected. For these conditions, "chance has a memory," meaning that the recurrence risk rises as the number of affected individuals within the family increases. If a family has multiple instances of a condition that is normally considered multifactorial, it is important to investigate the possibility of a single gene disorder.

Chromosomal Inheritance

A chromosome problem involves a missing or added segment of either a partial chromosome (such as a duplication or deletion) or a whole chromosome. Because

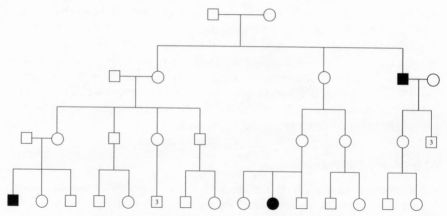

Figure 2.6 *Representative pedigree of multifactorial inheritance.*

the functions of multiple genes are disrupted, the affected individual usually has multiple problems including varying degrees of mental retardation. More than 600 chromosomal syndromes have been described (Connor and Ferguson-Smith, 1997).

There are several family and medical history clues that suggest a chromosomal problem (refer to Table 2.1). Always "think chromosomes" any time a child is born with three or more minor birth defects (such as protuberant ears, unusually shaped hands, and wide-spaced eyes). Minor anomalies are generally defined as characteristics that are of no serious cosmetic or functional consequence to the patient (Jones, 1997). A chromosome aberration should also be considered in an individual with two major defects (such as cleft lip and palate and a heart defect), or one major anomaly and two minor anomalies. Consider a chromosome study in any person with mental retardation, particularly if there are accompanying dysmorphic features or birth defects. A history of multiple miscarriages (three or more) is suggestive of a parental chromosome rearrangement. This is particularly true if there is a family history of multiple miscarriages and mental retardation, with or without associated birth defects (Fig. 2.7). A newborn with lymphedema may have an X chromosome monosomy or Trisomy 21. A karyotype to search for a sex chromosome anomaly should be considered in:

- An individual with ambiguous genitalia
- A fetus with cystic hygroma(s) (also common in trisomies 21 and 18)
- A newborn female with lymphedema
- A female with an inguinal hernia
- A female with primary amenorrhea
- A female with short stature and/or delayed or arrested puberty
- A male or female with failure to develop secondary sexual characteristics
- A male with hypogonadism and/or significant gynecomastia

The mental delay associated with chromosome problems is not regressive. Al-

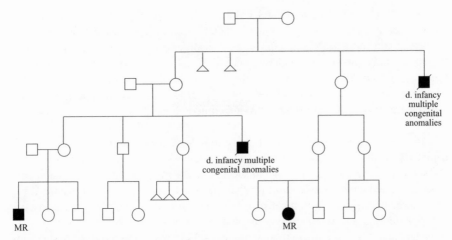

Figure 2.7 *Representative pedigree of an inherited chromosome translocation. Note the history of multiple miscarriages and individuals with mental retardation and multiple congenital anomalies.*

though a child with a chromosome anomaly may be born with serious medical problems, including mental retardation, he or she usually slowly advances to some ultimate level of functioning (albeit this level is usually below the average).

Changes in chromosome number are attributable to errors in meiosis (non-disjunction), resulting in trisomy (such as trisomy 18, or trisomy 21) or monosomy (such as the single X in Turner syndrome). These numerical chromosome errors are much more common than structural chromosomal changes (translocations). Most individuals with a chromosome anomaly will have an unremarkable family history.

The recurrence risk to have another child with a chromosome anomaly depends on the etiology of the chromosome anomaly. For example, the risk for a couple to have another child with a non-disjunctional chromosome anomaly is 1%, or the maternal age-related risk (whichever is higher). If a parent is a carrier for a structural chromosome translocation, the recurrence risk depends on the size of the rearrangement, the chromosomes involved, and which parent is a carrier. The risks when the mother carries the chromosome rearrangement are often higher than when the father is the carrier. Large unbalanced chromosome rearrangements may be lethal early in pregnancy. Most hereditary chromosome translocations have a recurrence risk for the parents of between 1 and 15%, although some hereditary chromosomal rearrangements are associated with much higher risks.

NONTRADITIONAL INHERITANCE PATTERNS

Triplet Repeat Disorders and the Inheritance of Dynamic Mutations

Anticipation describes the clinical phenomenon in which a genetic condition seems to worsen over successive generations. For example, a child with myotonic dystrophy may have severe hypotonia and failure to thrive, yet the affected grandparent has only early balding and pre-senile cataracts. Anticipation has mostly been described in autosomal dominant neurological disorders, such as Huntington disease, the spinocerebellar ataxias, and myotonic dystrophy (La Spada et al., 1994). In these conditions, nucleotide runs of three are excessively repeated in the DNA. Thus, they are called *trinucleotide* or *triplet repeat disorders*. Spinobulbar muscular atrophy and fragile X syndrome are X-linked neurological trinucleotide repeat disorders.

Most genes are transmitted unaltered through each generation of a family. In triplet repeat disorders, the triplet repeat is unstable once it reaches a critical size threshold, and the size can increase in successive generations. These unstable mutations are called *dynamic mutations* (Sutherland and Richards, 1994). It is normal to have fewer than a certain number of these trinucleotide repeats. The instability of the trinucleotide repeats tends to be related to their size (with longer repeats being more unstable and more likely to increase in size). Although contractions in size can occur, this is rare, and the contractions are usually small (less than five repeats) (La Spada et al., 1994). Some repeats are transmitted unchanged with neither expansion nor contraction.

A *premutation* describes an intermediate size range between trinucleotide repeat sizes in the normal (stable) range, and larger repeats in the range associated with disease. Individuals who carry a premutation often have no symptoms of disease, mild symptoms, or a later age of presentation of symptoms than individuals with larger expansions. Premutations are unstable and may expand into the full mutation range during meiosis.

For some trinucleotide repeat diseases, the stability of the mutation is influenced by the sex of the parent transmitting the mutation. Congenital myotonic dystrophy seems to be inherited exclusively from the mother, whereas childhood-onset Huntington disease seems to be inherited exclusively from the father. In fragile X syndrome, normal premutation carrier males cannot transmit a full mutation to their daughters, though all their daughters inherit the premutation. However, when the unstable fragile X mutation is transmitted by females, it usually increases in size (Nance, 1997a).

A large number of trinucleotide repeats is often associated with a more severe presentation of the disease (La Spada et al., 1994; Nance, 1997a). For example, in myotonic dystrophy, it is normal to have 30 or fewer CTG repeats. In the premutation range between 30 and 50 repeats, the individual is unlikely to develop symptoms of myotonic dystrophy. However, an expansion can occur in the egg or sperm of an unaffected premutation carrier; thus the person's offspring are at risk to be affected. An individual with a thousand or more CTG repeats usually displays the severe congenital form of myotonic dystrophy (Harper, 1997).

Huntington disease (HD) is an example of an autosomal dominant trinucleotide repeat disorder showing variable expressivity, age-related penetrance, anticipation, and parental bias in the stability of the trinucleotide repeat. Huntington disease is a progressive neurological condition characterized by uncontrolled movements (chorea) and problems with thinking, coordination and judgment. The penetrance is believed to be 90% by the age of 90, with an average age of symptom onset of 39 years (Nance, 1997a). The gene alteration in HD is a CAG repeat on the tip of the short arm of chromosome 4. An affected individual has 40 or more CAG repeats; an unaffected individual has 35 or fewer repeats. The area between 36 and 39 CAG repeats is considered an area of reduced penetrance (although the empirical penetrance risk is unknown) (ACMG/ASHG, 1998). Persons with repeat sizes in this range may or may not develop symptoms later in life. In the premutation range between 27 and 35 repeats, the individual will not be affected but an expansion can occur in the sperm (Brinkman, 1997; ACMG/ASHG, 1998). Juvenile Huntington disease is associated with CAG expansions over 80 repeats. These large expansions seem to be inherited exclusively from an affected father (Nance, 1997b).

Mitochondrial Inheritance

When P. D. Eastman penned the classic children's book *Are You My Mother?*, little did he realize that he had discovered the mantra of mitochondrial geneticists! Disorders caused by mitochondrial mutations have an unusual pedigree pattern—both males and females are affected, but the disease is transmitted exclusively through females (Fig. 2.8). There appears to be a random distribution of affected children. The expression of the disease is quite variable, both between families and within a family.

Within each cell, the number of mtDNA that carry the mutation vary. All the mtDNA within the mitochondrion may carry the mutation (*homoplasmy*), or only a fraction of the cellular mtDNA may be mutated (*heteroplasmy*). There is a threshold effect where a certain proportion of mutant mitochondria within a cell are tolerated (no disease). Severe disease is manifested when the proportion of mutant mitochondria is very high. Thus recurrence risk for the condition ranges from zero to 100%!

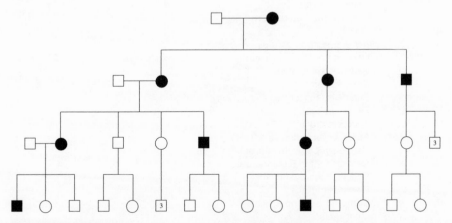

Figure 2.8 Representative pedigree of mitochondrial inheritance. Note that males and females are affected and that the condition is passed only through females. Usually there is great variability in the disease manifestations.

It is easy to confuse mitochondrial diseases and mitochondrial mutations. Genes within the nucleus (nuclear DNA) code for the majority of mitochondrial proteins, including the subunits of proteins involved in electron transport (oxidative phosphorylation). Mutations in these nuclear genes can be inherited in classic Mendelian patterns (autosomal recessive, autosomal dominant, or X-linked). Many mitochondrial disorders controlled by mutations in nuclear DNA have been identified. The mtDNA contains genes that code for the production of ribosomal RNA and various tRNAs necessary for mitochondrial protein biosynthesis, as well as some of the proteins involved in mitochondrial electron transport.

Mitochondria are important for energy production, specifically in their role in oxidative phosphorylation. Certain tissues and body organs depend more on mitochondrial energy metabolism than others. Mitochondrial diseases are most often associated with disorders of the central nervous system, the heart, skeletal muscle, endocrine glands, and kidneys (Wallace et al., 1997). Some of the clinical features of mitochondrial diseases are listed in Table 2.5. When taking a family history where a mitochondrial disorder is suspected, it is important to note all medical problems in family members. Because so many organ systems can be involved, even a seemingly insignificant medical problem may be related. Examples of common conditions caused by mitochondrial mutations are shown in Table 2.6.

Our understanding of mitochondrial diseases and mitochondrial inheritance is at the brink of explosion. Slightly more than 20 diseases have been linked to mito-

TABLE 2.5   Medical and Family History Features Suggestive of Conditions Caused by Mitochondrial Mutations

Frequent Features
   Persistent lactic acidosis
   Progressive or intermittent muscle weakness
   Hypotonia
   Failure to thrive
   Psychomotor retardation
   Seizures
Other Suggestive Features
   Oculomotor abnormalities, including ophthalmoplegia
   Retinal degeneration
   Optic atrophy
   Deafness (sensorineural)
   Slurred speech
   Short stature
   Apnea or tachypnea (periodic)
   Cardiomyopathy (hypertrophic)
   Cardiac rhythm disturbances
   Renal tubular dysfunction
   Diabetes mellitus
   Stroke (at a young age)
   Myoclonus
   Ataxia (progressive or intermittent)

Source: Adapted with permission from Clarke, 1996.

TABLE 2.6   Examples of Conditions with Mitochondrial Inheritance

Syndrome	Features
Kearns–Sayres syndrome (KSS)	Ophthalmoplegia (paralysis of the extraocular eye muscles) and retinal degeneration (usually before age 20 years), cerebellar dysfunction, psychomotor regression, ataxia, seizures, sensorineural deafness, cardiac conduction defects, short stature, lactic acidosis
MERRF (mitochondrial encephalomyopathy with ragged-red fibers)	Ataxia, spasticity, psychomotor regression, myoclonic seizures, sensorineural hearing loss, short stature, diabetes, lactic acidosis, lipomas (neck)
MELAS (mitochondrial encephalomyopathy, lactic acidosis, and strokes)	Bilateral cataracts, cortical blindness, ataxia, intermittent migraine headaches, seizures, myoclonus, sensorineural deafness, stroke-like episodes, myopathy, renal tubular dysfunction, cardiac conduction defects, short stature, diabetes mellitus, lactic acidosis
Neuropathy with ataxia and retinitis pigmentosa (NARP)	Retinitis pigmentosa, ataxia, sensory neuropathy, proximal muscle weakness, developmental delay, seizures, dementia, diabetes mellitus (occasional), lactic acidosis (occasional)
Leber hereditary optic neuropathy (LHON)	Midlife onset of optic atrophy (sudden central vision loss), cerebellar dysfunction (dystonia), and cardiac conduction defects
Chronic progressive external ophthalmoplegia (CPEO)	Progressive ophthalmoplegia, ptosis (droopy eyelids)
Diabetes mellitus type II and sensorineural hearing loss	Several families have been described with mitochondrial mutations

Sources: Clarke, 1996; OMIM, 1998; Wallace et al., 1997.

chondrial inheritance. Mitochondrial inheritance has been implicated for some manifestations of common diseases such as nonsyndromic hearing loss, stroke, epilepsy, and diabetes mellitus (Wallace et al., 1997). The recognition of mitochondrial inheritance patterns will undoubtedly play an increasingly important role in the evolving clinical realm of genomic medicine.

Contiguous Gene Syndromes

If the affected individual has multiple systems or organs involved (*pleiotropy*), this may be a *contiguous gene syndrome* (CGS). This terminology describes a loss of chromosomal material resulting in disruption of function in several genes located in a row. Specifically, they affect normal gene dosage (Ledbetter and Ballabio, 1995). These are submicroscopic deletions or duplications of multiple unrelated genes that are located next to each other at a specific chromosome locus that each independently contribute to the phenotype. For example, neurofibromatosis is an autosomal dominant syndrome characterized by multiple café au lait spots and neurofibromas. Rarely this syndrome is also associated with mental retardation and dysmorphic features. It is now known that this association represents a contiguous gene syndrome (Kayes et al., 1994).

Contiguous gene syndromes have played an important role in the isolation and localization of disease genes. For example, in 1985 Francke and colleagues described a boy with Duchenne muscular dystrophy, chronic granulomatous disease, retinitis pigmentosa, and McLeod syndrome who was missing a segment of chromosomal material at Xp21 (Francke et al., 1985). This finding led to the discovery of gene alterations for all the aforementioned syndromes. Individuals with schizophrenia, mental retardation, and dysmorphic features have been identified as having microdeletion contiguous gene syndromes. The study of such syndromes is helping researchers define genetic loci for complex conditions such as schizophrenia (Bennett et al., 1997; Karayiorgou and Gogos, 1997).

The availability of FISH (fluorescence in situ hybridization), a technique of using molecular probes to visualize minute chromosomal changes, provides powerful and sensitive diagnostic testing for contiguous gene syndromes.

Imprinting

Imprinting refers to the modification of a gene (or a chromosomal region) such that it is expressed differently if it is inherited from one parent versus the other parent. The imprinted copy of the gene is inactivated; therefore it is not expressed. The imprint is reversible because a man passes on his genes with his own paternal imprint if those genes were inherited with a maternal imprint from his mother (Strachan and Read, 1996). The mechanism of imprinting appears to involve DNA methylation (the modification of DNA by the addition of a methyl group), but the details are complex and are poorly understood (Strachan and Read, 1996). Imprinting appears to occur at the level of transcription, most likely in the germ line, or in the early zygote before the male and female pronuclei fuse (Strachan and Read, 1996). It is unclear whether or not imprinting is a critical process in embryonic development and the expression of genetic disease or a property of a limited number of genes (or small chromosomal regions). Most genes are not subject to imprinting or we would not so readily recognize simple Mendelian inheritance patterns. Imprinting, or rather the lack of imprinting (termed loss of imprinting or LOI), may play an important role in the abnormal gene expression patterns in human tumor cell growth. (Feinberg, 1998). A current map of imprinted human chromosomes can be viewed at http://www.genes.uchicago.edu.

Classic examples of imprinting are Prader–Willi syndrome and Angelman syndrome. Both of these distinctly different genetic conditions have alterations in the same genetic region—a tiny segment of the long arm (q arm) of chromosome 15 (15q11-q13). If the altered region is inherited from the father, the child (son or daughter) has Prader–Willi syndrome. The hallmark features of Prader–Willi syndrome are hypotonia in childhood, almond-shaped eyes, small hands and feet, obesity and overeating, and a mean IQ of 50. If the same altered region is inherited from the mother, the child (son or daughter) has Angelman syndrome. Severe developmental delay, limited speech, jerky movements, hysterical laughter, and an unusual facial appearance characterize Angelman syndrome (Sapienza and Hall, 1995).

Providing genetic counseling and risk assessment for families with Angelman syndrome or Prader–Willi syndrome is complicated, and requires a careful family history and sophisticated genetic testing. To date, six genetic classes of Angelman syndrome have been identified (Stalker and Williams, 1998). The majority of patients (about 70%) have large deletions of the maternal 15q11–q13 region. The recurrence risk for the parents of these individuals is less than 1%. A small percentage of individuals with Angelman syndrome and Prader–Willi syndrome are thought to have mutations in an imprinting control center that controls imprinting and gene expression via methylation and demethylation in the 15q11–q13 region (Stalker and Williams, 1998). In other instances, the mother can carry a mutation in UBE3A (a ubiquitin-protein ligase). In the latter two circumstances, the mother would have as much as a 50% recurrence risk for future pregnancies (as would her female relatives who carry the mutation). Male relatives who carry either of these mutations would not be at risk to have affected children, but might have affected grandchildren through their daughters (Malzac et al., 1998; Stalker and Williams, 1998).

Uniparental Disomy

This is a recently recognized phenomenon whereby an individual receives both copies of a specific chromosome from one parent and no copy from the other parent. Thus far uniparental disomy (UPD) has been documented for more than 13 of the 22 autosomes, both X chromosomes and the XY pair (Engel, 1995; Engel, 1998). Several genetic conditions have been described in which UPD has been observed. For example, a few individuals with classic autosomal recessive cystic fibrosis have inherited both chromosomes with the cystic fibrosis mutation from one parent (the other parent has two normal alleles) (Cutting, 1997). Uniparental disomy has been observed in 2–3% of individuals with Angelman syndrome where the child inherits two critical regions of chromosome 15 from the father. The opposite has also occurred, where a child inherits two chromosome 15s from the mother and thus has Prader–Willi syndrome (Malzac et al., 1998; Stalker and Williams, 1998).

For some chromosomes, uniparental disomy may produce no effect, and for other chromosomes it may be lethal (Strachan and Read, 1996; Engel, 1998; Field et al., 1998). Uniparental disomy can cause morbidity or lethality by altering imprinting processes, mimicking disease deletions or duplications, generating recessive disorders when only one parent is a carrier, or prompting malignant tumor development (Engel, 1995). Although misattribution of paternity is the most likely explanation if a child with a classic autosomal recessive condition has only one parent who is a carrier, uniparental disomy should be a consideration.

OTHER FACTORS TO CONSIDER

New Hereditary Mutations

Many autosomal dominant, X-linked recessive, and mitochondrially inherited conditions have a high new mutation rate. This means that the affected person is the first person in the family to have the condition. The mutation occurred in the egg or sperm that "created" that person. All of the daughter cells from the fertilized egg carry the alteration, including the gonads. The affected individual has a chance to pass the mutation on to his or her children. The siblings and parents of that affected individual do not have an increased chance to have a child with the same condition.

Mosaicism

Mosaicism describes the phenomenon when some cells in an organ or tissue have a different genetic constitution from the other cells. *Chromosomal mosaicism* refers to a chromosome abnormality that occurs after fertilization during mitosis at an early cell stage. For example, a child who has mosaic trisomy 21 (Down syndrome) has some cells that are normal (diploid), and some cells that have the extra 21st chromosome (trisomy).

If the cells in the gonads (testes and ovaries) are mosaic, this is called *gonadal mosaicism*. The risk to have an affected child depends on the percentage of gonadal involvement. Recurrence risk ranges from 0 to 50%. In *somatic mosaicism* there is no increased risk for affected offspring, because the mutation is not in the gonads. Somatic mosaicism occurs in tumor cells—some cells in the body contain an altered chromosome or single gene mutation, whereas others do not. It is interesting to note that somatic mitochondrial mutations accumulate in all cells with age. It is hypothesized that these mitochondrial mutations may play a role in late-onset degenerative diseases and aging (Wallace et al., 1997).

Sporadic Conditions

Inheritance of a condition is described as "sporadic" when the parents' risk to have another child with the condition is considered negligible (in the range of less than 1%). These conditions are often severe and the affected child does not reproduce. As we learn more about genetic mechanisms, some of these conditions are now known to be a result of contiguous gene syndromes, gonadal mosaicism in one of the parents, or new autosomal dominant or X-linked mutations. In these instances, the parents of the affected child may have a risk for recurrence. The affected individual may have as much as a 50:50 chance to have an affected son or daughter if he or she carries a new dominant mutation. Usually the healthy siblings of the affected individual have a low risk of having affected children.

Environmental Factors

In taking a genetic family history, it is important to remember the role that the environment plays in gene expression. For example, a history of two sisters dying of lung cancer is much more worrisome if the sisters never smoked cigarettes than if they each smoked a pack of cigarettes a day for 20 years. The contribution of environmental factors to gene expression will continue to be elucidated as more genes are identified for common genetic disorders.

SUMMARY

The patterns of Mendel have been genetic dogma since the turn of the 20th century. Health professionals must be receptive to new ways of thinking about human inheritance. Forty years ago genetic doctrine was rocked by the recognition that a human cell has 46 chromosomes, not 48. The past 10 years mark the discovery of entirely new inheritance patterns such as mitochondrial inheritance, imprinting, and dynamic mutations. The family pedigree will undoubtedly serve as a template for new discoveries in gene action and interaction as the practice of genomic medicine unfolds.

REFERENCES

American College of Medical Genetics/American Society of Human Genetics (ACMG/ASHG) Huntington Disease Genetic Testing Working Group (1998). Laboratory guidelines for Huntington disease genetic testing. Am J Hum Genet 62:1243–1247.

Bennett RL, Karayiorgou M, Sobin CA, Norwood TH, Kay MA (1997). Identification of an interstitial deletion in an adult female with schizophrenia, mental retardation, and dysmorphic features: further support for a putative schizophrenia-susceptibility locus at 5q21-23.1. Am J Hum Genet 61(6):1450–1454.

Brinkman RR, Mezei MM, Theilmann J, Almqvist E, Hayden MR (1997). The likelihood of being affected with Huntington disease by a particular age, for a specific CAG size. Am J Hum Genet 60(5):1202–1210.

Clarke JTR (1996). *A Clinical Guide to Inherited Metabolic Diseases*. Great Britain: Cambridge University Press.

Connor M, Ferguson-Smith M (1997). *Essential Medical Genetics*, 5th ed. Oxford: Blackwell Scientific.

Cutting GR (1997). Cystic fibrosis. In Rimoin DL, Connor JM, Pyeritz RE (eds), *Emory and Rimoin's Principles and Practice of Medical Genetics*, 3rd ed. New York: Churchill Livingstone, pp. 2685–2717.

DePasquale SE, Giordano A, Donnenfeld AE (1998). The genetics of ovarian cancer: molecular biology and clinical application. Obstet Gynecol Surv 53(4):248–256.

Emery AEH (1997). Duchenne and other X-linked muscular dystrophies. In Rimoin DL,

Connor JM, Pyeritz RE (eds), *Emory and Rimoin's Principles and Practice of Medical Genetics*, 3rd ed. New York: Churchill Livingstone, pp. 2337–2354.

Engel E (1995). Uniparental disomy: a review of causes and clinical sequelae. Ann Genet 38(3):113–136.

Engel E (1998). Uniparental disomies in unselected populations. Am J Hum Genet 63:962–966.

Feinberg AP (1998). Genomic imprinting and cancer. In Vogelstein B, Kinzler KW (eds), *The Genetic Basis of Human Cancer*. New York: McGraw-Hill, pp. 95–107.

Field LL, Tobias R, Robinson WP et al. (1998). Maternal uniparental disomy of chromosome 1 with no apparent phenotypic effects. Am J Hum Genet 63:1216–1220.

Francke U, Ochs HD, De Martinville B et al. (1985). Minor Xp21 chromosome deletion in a male associated with expression of Duchenne muscular dystrophy, chronic granulomatous disease, retinitis pigmentosa, and McLeod syndrome. Am J Hum Genet 37:250.

Gorlin RJ, Cohen MM, Levin LS (1990). *Syndromes of the Head and Neck*, 3rd ed. New York: Oxford University Press.

Harper PS (1997). Myotonic dystrophy. In Rimoin DL, Connor JM, Pyeritz RE (eds), *Emory and Rimoin's Principles and Practice of Medical Genetics*, 3rd ed. New York: Churchill Livingstone, pp. 2425–2443.

Houlston R, Bourne TH, Davies A, et al. (1992). Use of family history in a screening clinic for familial ovarian cancer. Gynecol Oncol 47:247–252.

Jones KL (1997). *Smith's Recognizable Patterns of Human Malformation*, 5th ed. Philadelphia: WB Saunders Co.

Karayiorgou M, Gogos JA (1997). Dissecting the genetic complexity of schizophrenia. Mol Psychiatry 2(3):211–223.

Kayes LM, Burke W, Riccardi VM, et al. (1994). Deletions spanning the neurofibromatosis 1 gene: identification and phenotype of five patients. Am J Hum Genet 54(3):424–436.

La Spada AR, Paulson HL, Fishbeck KH (1994). Trinucleotide repeat expansion in neurological disease. Ann Neurol 36:814–822.

Ledbetter DH, Ballabio A (1995). Molecular cytogenetics of contiguous gene syndromes: mechanisms and consequences of gene dosage imbalance. In Scriver CR, Beaudet AL, Sly WS, Valle D (eds), *The Metabolic and Molecular Bases of Inherited Disease*. New York: McGraw-Hill, pp. 811–839.

Malzac P, Webber H, Moncla A, et al. (1998). Mutation analysis in UBE3A in Angelman syndrome patients. Am J Hum Genet 52:1353–1360.

Nance MA (1997a). Clinical aspects of CAG repeat diseases. Brain Pathol 7(3):881–900.

Nance MA (1997b). Genetic testing of children at risk for Huntington's disease. US Huntington Disease Genetic Testing Group. Neurology 49(4):1048–1053.

NIH Consensus Statement (1997 Apr 14–16). Genetic Testing for Cystic Fibrosis. 15(4):1–37.

Offit K (1998). *Clinical Cancer Genetics: Risk Counseling and Management*. New York: John Wiley and Sons.

Okabe M, Ikawa M, Ashkenas J (1998). Male infertility and the genetics of spermatogenesis. Am J Hum Genet 62:1274–1281.

Online Mendelian Inheritance in Man, OMIM ™. Center for Medical Genetics, Johns Hopkins University (Baltimore, MD) and National Center for Biotechnology Information, National Library of Medicine (Bethesda, MD), 1997. Accessed June 19, 1998. World Wide Web URL:http://www.ncbi.nlm.nih.gov/omim/

Reeves WB, Andreoli TE (1995). Nephrogenic diabetes insipidus. In Scriver CR, Beaudet AL, Sly WS, Valle D (eds), *The Metabolic and Molecular Bases of Inherited Disease.* New York: McGraw-Hill, pp. 3045–3071.

Rimoin DL, Connor JM, Pyeritz RE (eds) (1997). *Emory and Rimoin's Principles and Practice of Medical Genetics*, 3rd ed. New York: Churchill Livingstone.

Robinson A, Linden MG (1993). *Clinical Genetics Handbook.* Boston: Blackwell Scientific Publications.

Sapienzia C, Hall JG (1995). Genetic imprinting in human disease. In Scriver CR, Beaudet AL, Sly WS, Valle D (eds), *The Metabolic and Molecular Bases of Inherited Disease.* New York: McGraw-Hill, pp. 437–458.

Scriver CR, Beaudet AL, Sly WS, Valle D (eds) (1995). *The Metabolic and Molecular Bases of Inherited Disease*, 7th ed. New York: McGraw-Hill.

Stalker HJ, Williams CA (1998). Genetic counseling in Angelman syndrome: the challenges of multiple causes. Am J Med Genet 77:54–59.

Strachan T, Read AP (1996). *Human Molecular Genetics.* New York: Wiley-Liss.

Sutherland GR, Richards RI (1994). Dynamic mutations. Am Scientist 82:157–163.

Sybert VP (1997). *Genetic Skin Disorders.* New York, Oxford: Oxford University Press.

Vogel F, Motulsky AG (1996). *Human Genetics: Problems and Approaches*, 3rd ed. Berlin: Springer.

Wallace DC, Brown MD, Lott MR (1997). Mitochondrial genetics. In Rimoin DL, Connor JM, Pyeritz RE (eds), *Principles and Practice of Medical Genetics*, 3rd ed. New York: Churchill Livingstone, pp. 277–322.

3

Getting to the Roots: Recording the Family Tree

A complete pedigree is often a work of great labour, and in its finished form is frequently a work of art.
—***Karl Pearson, 1912 (from Resta, 1993)***

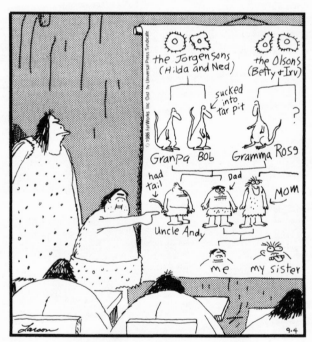

Dirk brings his family tree to class

CREATING A MEDICAL PEDIGREE: GETTING STARTED

The basic medical pedigree is a graphic depiction of how family members are biologically and legally related to one another, from one generation to the next. Each family member is represented by a square (male), or a circle (female), and they are connected to each other by relationship lines. This family "map" is meaningless if the symbols cannot be interpreted from clinician to clinician. The symbols outlined here are from the 1995 recommendations of the National Society of Genetic Counselors Pedigree Standardization Task Force (Bennett et al., 1995). For personal use, you may photocopy Appendix A.1 for a handy, double-sided "cheat sheet" containing common pedigree symbols, the basic information to include on a pedigree, and a prototype imaginary pedigree using all the standardized symbols. The pedigree icons in and of themselves provide scant information; the power of a pedigree lies within the associative network of symbols.

Generally, the pedigree is taken in a face-to-face interview with the patient, before the physical examination. A patient is usually more comfortable sharing the intimate details of his or her personal and family life while fully clothed rather than wearing one of the highly fashionable rear-exposure gowns that are available in most examination rooms.

I find it useful to take a preliminary pedigree on the telephone. Many patients have limited knowledge of the health of their extended relatives. By asking medical-family history questions in advance of the appointment, the patient can do the homework of contacting the appropriate family members to get more accurate details. The patient can also help to arrange to obtain medical records (see Chapter 6). At the appointment, the pedigree that was taken by telephone can be verified with the patient. Medical-family history questionnaires can be a useful tool to collect pertinent information before the patient's appointment. However, a questionnaire should not substitute for an actual pedigree. Sample genetic family history questionnaires for cancer and a child being placed for adoption are included in Appendices A.3 and A.4, respectively.

The *consultand* is the individual seeking genetic counseling and/or testing . This person is identified on the pedigree by an arrow, so that he or she can be easily identified when referring to the pedigree. If more than one person (consultands) come to the appointment (for example, a parent and child, or two sisters), identify each person with an arrow on the pedigree. The consultand can be a healthy person or a person with a medical condition.

The *proband* is the *affected* individual that brings the family to medical attention (Marazita, 1995). Identifying the proband is important in genetic mapping studies and research. Some researchers use the term propositus (plural is propositi) interchangeably with proband(s). The *index case* is a term used in genetic research to describe the first affected person to be studied in the family. Sometimes an individual is both a proband and the consultand.

Even with the use of standardized pedigree symbols, a *key* or *legend* is essential for any pedigree. The main purpose of the key is to define the shading (or hatching) of symbols that indicate who is affected on the pedigree. The key is also used to ex-

TABLE 3.1   Essential Information to Record on Family Members in a Pedigree

Age, birth date, or year of birth
Age at death (year if known)
Cause of death
Full sibs versus half sibs
Relevant health information (e.g., height, weight)
Age at diagnosis
Affected/unaffected status (define shading of symbol in key/legend)
Personally evaluated or medically documented (*)
Testing status ("E" is used for evaluation on pedigree and defined in key/legend)
Pregnancies with gestational age noted LMP or EDD (estimated date of delivery)
Pregnancy complications with gestational age noted (e.g., 6 wk, 34 wk): miscarriage (SAB),
   stillbirth (SB), pregnancy termination (TOP), ectopic (ECT)
Infertility vs. no children by choice
Ethnic background for each grandparent
Use a "?" if family history is unknown/unavailable
Consanguinity (note degree of relationship if not implicit in pedigree)
Family names (if appropriate)
Date pedigree taken or updated
Name of person who took pedigree, and credentials (M.D., R.N., M.S., C.G.C.)
Key/legend

plain any infrequently used symbols (such as adoption or artificial insemination) or uncommon abbreviations.

Table 3.1 serves as a quick reference to the information essential to record on a pedigree. Remember to document on the pedigree your name and credentials (such as R.N., M.D., M.S.), and the name of the consultand (the person who has the appointment). It is also helpful to record the name of the *historian* (the person giving the information). For example, a foster or adoptive parent may not have access to accurate history about the biological family of the child. Remember to date the pedigree. This is particularly important if ages rather than birth dates are recorded for family members on the pedigree. Was the pedigree taken yesterday or 10 years ago?

Use abbreviations sparingly and define them in the key. For example, CP may be short for cleft palate or cerebral palsy; MVA may mean motor vehicle accident or multiple vascular accidents; SB may be interpreted as stillbirth, spina bifida, or even shortness of breath!

Because the pedigree is part of the patient's medical record, it should be drawn with permanent ink. Using a black pen is best because blue ink may be faint if the record is microfilmed. It is acceptable to draft a pedigree in pencil; just be wary of errors in transcription. My favorite pedigree drawing tool is a correction pen that quickly obliterates my frequent drawing errors.

Draw the pedigree on your institution's medical progress notepaper (if available). A sample pedigree form is included for your use in Appendix A.2. A standardized pedigree form has the advantage that you can include common pedigree symbols as a reference on the form. This fill-in-the-blanks approach serves as a reminder to document easily overlooked family history information (such as family ethnicity and whether or not there is consanguinity). These forms are limited in that pedigrees of large families may be difficult to squeeze onto the page.

Plastic drawing templates of various-sized circles, squares, triangles, diamonds, and arrows, are helpful for keeping the pedigree symbols neat and of uniform size. Such templates are available at most art and office supply stores.

Computer software programs for drawing pedigrees are reviewed in Appendix A.5: The Genetics Library. Most of the currently available programs are not practical for drawing a quick pedigree in a clinical setting. These drawing programs are efficacious for large research pedigrees, patient registries, or in preparing a pedigree for professional publication.

Laying The Foundation—Pedigree Line Definitions

Pedigrees can become quite complicated when they include multiple generations. Add to this the common occurrence of a person having children with multiple partners, and a pedigree soon looks like a television-wiring diagram! There are four main "line definitions" which form the "trunk" and "branches" of a medical family tree (Fig. 3.1). Here are some simple rules to remember:

- A *relationship line* is a horizontal line between two partners; a slash or break in this line documents a separation or divorce.
- If possible, the male partner should be to the left of the female partner. (See Chapter 8, Fig. 8.1 for how to draw relationships between same-sex partners.)
- A couple who is *consanguineous* (meaning they are biological relatives such as cousins) should be connected by a *double* relationship line (Figs. 3.10 and 3.11).

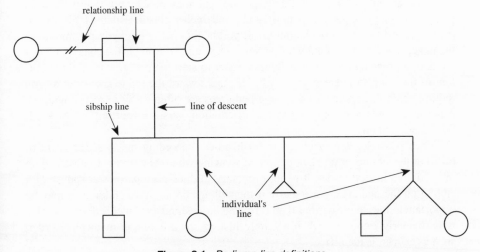

Figure 3.1   *Pedigree line definitions.*

- The *sibship line* is a horizontal line connecting brothers and sisters ("sibs").
- Each sibling has a vertical *individual's line* attached to the horizontal sibship line.
- *Twins* (fraternal/dizygotic or identical/monozygotic) share one vertical individual's line, attached to the horizontal sibship line.
- For pregnancies not carried to term, the individual's line is shorter (Fig. 3.5).
- The *line of descent* is a vertical bridge connecting the horizontal sibship line to the horizontal relationship line.

Remembering the applications of these line definitions is important in the pedigree symbolization of adoption (Fig. 3.7), and in symbolizing assisted reproductive technologies or ART (see Chapter 8 and Fig. 8.1).

Keeping Track of Who is Who on the Pedigree

Begin by asking the consultand (or a parent if the consultand is a child):

"Do you have a partner, or are you married?"
"How many biological brothers and sisters do you have?"
"How many children do you have?"

The answers to these questions give you an idea of how much room you will need on the paper to draw the pedigree.

Always ask if siblings share the same mother and father—people often do not distinguish an adopted sibling or a stepsibling from biological kin. Remind the historian that you are also interested in information about deceased relatives. For example, an adult may forget to tell you about a sibling who died as an infant 25 years ago.

If you are interviewing an elderly person, you may be taking a five-generation pedigree (e.g., grandparents, parents, aunts and uncles, cousins, siblings, nieces and nephews, children and grandchildren). If you begin your pedigree in the middle of the page, it is easy to extend your pedigree "up" and "down." If the consultand is a child, or a pregnant mother, usually it is easier to start the pedigree toward the bottom of the page and extend your pedigree "up" toward the top of the paper as you inquire about prior generations. Large pedigrees are often easier to record with the paper in a "landscape" or "lengthwise" orientation, versus a "portrait" or "up-and-down" orientation.

When possible, draw siblings in birth order. Recording the ages (or years of birth) of the siblings is an obvious way of showing when they are *not* represented on the pedigree in birth order. It is not necessary to draw each partner or spouse of a sibling on the pedigree, particularly if the siblings do not have children. It may be important to record the partner if an offspring has a significant medical history. This is particularly important when a family history for a common medical disorder, such as cancer, is identified.

Each generation in a pedigree should be on the same horizontal plane. For example, a person's siblings and cousins are drawn on the same horizontal axis; the parents, aunts, and uncles are drawn on the same horizontal line. In pedigrees used for publication or research, usually each generation is defined by a Roman numeral (e.g., I, II, III), and each person in the generation is given an Arabic number, from left to right (e.g., I-3, I-4, II-3). This makes it easy to refer to family members in the pedigree by number, and thus protects family confidentiality (Fig. 3.2). In clinical pedigrees, names are usually recorded on the pedigree (parallel or next to the individual's line). The family surname is placed above the sibship line, or above the relationship line. Of course, if names are recorded on the pedigree, care must be taken to preserve the confidentiality of the pedigree.

How Many Generations Are Included In A Pedigree?

A basic pedigree usually includes three generations—the consultand's *first-degree relatives* (parents, children, siblings) and *second-degree relatives* (half siblings, grandparents, aunts and uncles, grandchildren). *Third-degree relatives*, particularly cousins, are often included, if only to note that they "exist." For example, one can place a diamond with a "3" inside to show that an aunt or uncle has three children. Figure 3.3 shows the pedigree framework for denoting a relative's relationship to the proband (for example, a first cousin is a third-degree relative to the proband).

If a health problem of significance is identified, the pedigree is extended back as far as possible (Refer to Table 4.1 for clues to family history features suggestive of a genetic disorder). For example, if a 60-year-old woman with breast cancer is interested in genetic risk assessment for her two daughters, you would ask her about any cancer in her parents, grandparents, uncles and aunts, cousins, children, and grandchildren. You would inquire about great-aunts and great-uncles and great-grandpar-

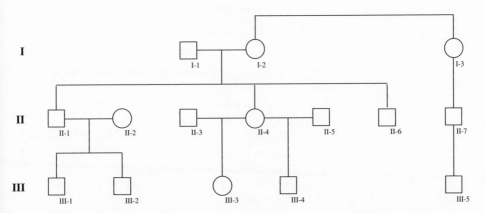

Figure 3.2 *Numbering generations and individuals on a pedigree. This numbering system allows for easy reference to individuals on a pedigree when names are not recorded.*

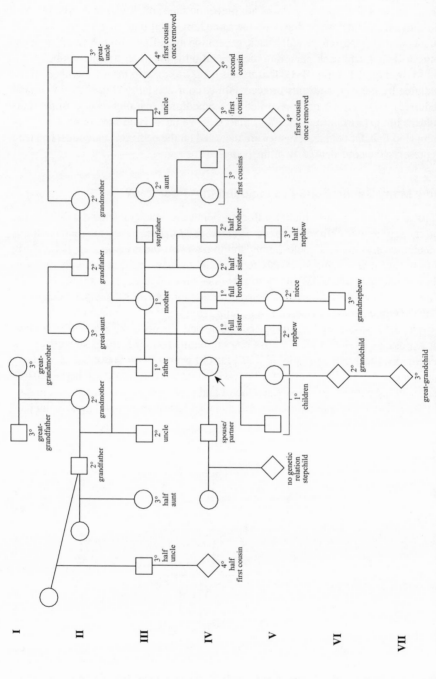

Figure 3.3 The pedigree framework for denoting a relative's relationship to the proband (i.e., first-degree, second-degree, and third-degree relatives).

ents if a positive family history were found. The pedigree for a genetic condition with a late age of symptom onset may be quite extensive.

THE BASIC PEDIGREE SYMBOLS

The most common pedigree symbols are shown in Figure 3.4. The gender of an individual is assigned by the outward phenotype. This is important when drawing a pedigree for a child with ambiguous genitalia. The age (or date of birth) is noted for each individual. Record the cause of death and age at death for all individuals on the pedigree. Noting the year of death is useful because this can provide you with clues as to the diagnostic tools available during that medical era. For example, DNA diagnostic testing did not exist before the mid-1980s. The identification of a structural brain anomaly may have been made with the aid of a pneumoencephalogram in the 1960s and 1970s, compared to the modern brain imaging techniques of computerized tomography (CT scans) or magnetic resonance imaging (MRI).

Relevant health information, such as height (h.) and weight (w.), is placed below the pedigree symbol. The recommended order of this information is as follows: (1) age, birth date, or year of birth; (2) age at death and cause; (3) relevant health information; and (4) pedigree number.

It is the rare historian who knows the precise details of such information as current ages, ages at death, and the heights of his or her extended family. A tilde (~) can be used when approximations are given.

Pedigree Symbols Related to Pregnancy and Reproduction

The various pedigree symbols related to pregnancy, spontaneous abortion, termination of pregnancy, stillbirth, and infertility are shown in Figure 3.5. Always include the gestational age, in weeks (wk), if known, below the symbol. An approximation of dates can be shown, such as "~12 wk." Usually the gestational age is stated as the date of the last menstrual period (LMP) or the estimated date of confinement (EDC). Some clinicians prefer using EDD (estimated date of delivery) because the description "confinement" seems archaic. You can note pregnancy dating by ultrasound (US) as "US 12 wk."

A stillbirth (SB) is defined as the "birth of a dead child with gestational age noted" (Bennett et al., 1995).

If the sex of the fetus is known, one can note male or female under the appropriate symbol. This is preferable to making the symbol a square or circle. If a chromosome study has confirmed the sex of the fetus, this can be noted under the symbol as "46,XX" or "46,XY."

Yours, Mine, and Ours—The Blended Family

Correct documentation of how individuals are biologically related to each other is essential for accurate pedigree assessment. It is almost inevitable when taking a

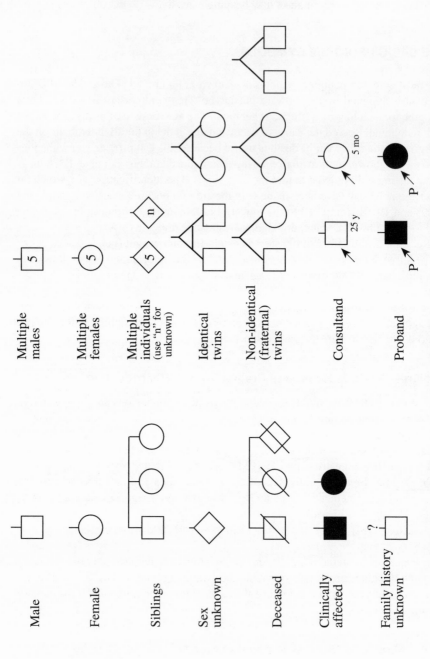

Figure 3.4 The most common pedigree symbols. Pregnancy-related symbols are shown in Figure 3.5.

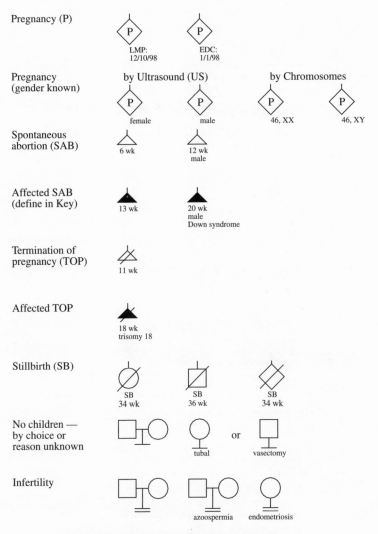

Figure 3.5 *Pedigree symbols related to pregnancy.*

family history that at least one person in the family will have more than one partner. For each sibling group in the pedigree, ask if they share the same mother and father. If the answer is "No," ask "Which of your brothers and sisters share the same mother, and which share the same father?"

If there is a big gap in ages between siblings, this is a clue that they may be half siblings. The gap may also be an indication of a period of infertility.

It is not necessary to include each partner of an individual on a pedigree, as is illustrated by actress Elizabeth Taylor's marriage history in Figure 3.6.

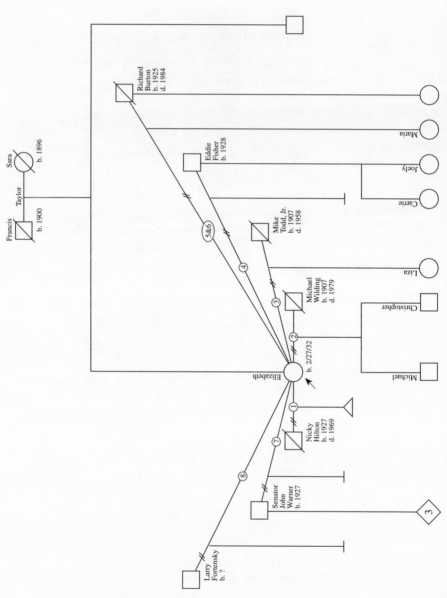

Figure 3.6 A pedigree of actress Elizabeth Taylor demonstrating how to illustrate multiple marriage partners, stepchildren, and half siblings. (Source: www.celebsite.com)

Adoption

It is important to distinguish a person who is adopted "in" to a family (nonbiological relative) from a person who is adopted "out" (a biological relative). For any adoption, brackets are placed on either side of the appropriate symbol for male, female, or sex-unknown (a diamond). If a person or couple adopts the person "in," the individual's line is dotted (indicating a nonbiological relationship). A person who is placed for adoption by birth parents has a solid individual's line.

It is not uncommon for a family member to adopt a relative (for example, a sibling adopting a niece or nephew, or grandparents adopting a grandchild). The method of recording this situation on a pedigree is shown in Figure 3.7.

When a person or couple adopts a child, it is useful to inquire if this was for a medical reason (such as an illness, a known genetic disease, or infertility in the adoptive parents). The reason can be noted below the line of descent.

When a child is placed for adoption, information about the child's medical her-

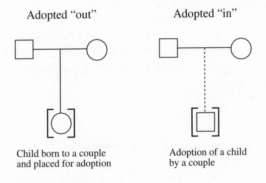

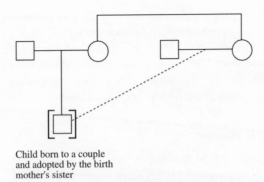

Figure 3.7 *Pedigree symbolization of adoption.*

itage is usually given to the new parents (See Chapter 7). A sample adoptive medical–family history form can be found in Appendix A.4.

Infertility Versus No Children By Choice

If a person (or couple) is of reproductive age and does not have children, inquire if this is by choice or for a biological reason. The cause of infertility should be noted below the individual's line (e.g., azoospermia, endometriosis) (Fig. 3.5).

Affected Status: Shading the Pedigree Symbols

Accurately documenting who is affected and unaffected on a pedigree is critical for pedigree analysis. A symbol should *only* be shaded in if the person (or pregnancy, miscarriage, etc.) is *clinically symptomatic* with the condition. Of course, this may be a function of the clinical "tool" that is used to define affected status. For example, the 2-year-old sister of a 5-year-old boy with classic symptoms of cystic fibrosis may have no detectable symptoms, yet have elevated sweat chloride levels.

Most families will have more than one genetic, or potentially heritable, medical condition. Different shading can be used to define the different diseases on the pedigree. For example, when documenting a family history of cancer, shading in the various quadrants of each square (male) or circle (female) is a way to symbolize multiple cancers (Fig. 3.8).

A&W

While seeing this abbreviation may cause you to salivate for your favorite root beer beverage, this is actually a simple method of showing on the pedigree that a family member is "alive and well." By noting "A&W" under each healthy person on the pedigree, you can be assured that you asked about the health of each member on the pedigree.

"He Died of A Broken Heart"—Family Hearsay

Family members often use nonmedical terms to describe illnesses in a family. If Uncle Billy "died of a broken heart," the clinician should not automatically assume that the person died of a heart attack. The family lore can be included on the pedigree in "quotes," using the words the historian used to describe the ailment. Asking questions such as, "Was this a long-standing illness or was the death unexpected?" might help to clarify the nature of the family member's illness.

Family History Unknown

Like the rogue in the 1970s Paul Simon tune, "Fifty Ways to Leave Your Lover," sometimes little information is known about a parent, grandparent, or other family member. Placing a question mark above the pedigree symbol shows that you in-

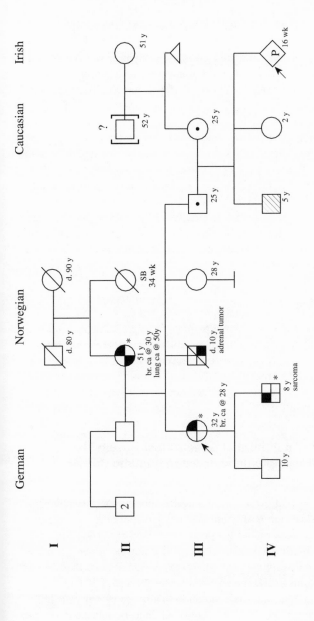

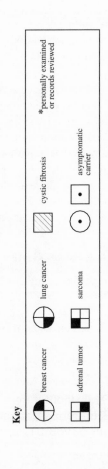

Figure 3.8 Hypothetical pedigree demonstrating how to shade affected individuals when more than one condition is segregating in a family.

quired about that individual's family history, but the information is unknown or unavailable (Fig. 3.4).

DOCUMENTING MEDICAL EXAMINATIONS AND EVALUATIONS

Genetic counseling requires accurate medical information. An asterisk (*) is placed near the lower right edge of the pedigree symbol for anyone who has been personally examined by you (or another team member), or if you have verified medical records (Fig. 3.9). See Chapter 6 for specific information on how to help families obtain medical records on family members.

Medical evaluations on family members can be recorded on the pedigree. Each clinical evaluation or test is represented by an "E" and defined in the key. An evaluation may represent information obtained by clinical examination, medical testing (e.g., brain imaging, nerve conduction studies), or molecular genetic test results. If a test or examination result is abnormal it is considered a "+" result, and a normal result is documented as "−." If the test is uninformative, a "u" follows the "E." For example, there are hundreds of mutations in the cystic fibrosis gene. A child with known cystic fibrosis may have only one mutation identified. This could be noted on the pedigree as ΔF508/u (Fig. 3.9).

A Note on Genetic Testing

Genetic testing confuses many patients. Some patients falsely assume any genetic test is a chromosome test. Others assume that all genetic tests involve direct analysis of the DNA (versus a linkage study or enzyme analysis). Patients also mistakenly think that when they have a DNA test, their DNA is screened for all genetic diseases. It is always important to obtain documentation of the patient's or family member's actual laboratory result.

The Healthy Person with An Abnormal Genetic Test Result: The Difference between a Presymptomatic or Asymptomatic Carrier and an Obligate Carrier

Advances in genetic testing now allow us to test a healthy person for a genetic condition that they may or will develop in the future. Many geneticists reserve the description *presymptomatic carrier* for a healthy person who is likely to develop a genetic disease in his or her lifetime (Bennett et al, 1995). For example, a healthy person at risk for Huntington disease who has a CAG expansion of more than 40 repeats is likely to have symptoms of HD if he or she reaches the age of 70 (Brinkman et al., 1997). In contrast, a woman who has a mutation in a breast cancer gene has a higher lifetime risk to develop breast and possibly other cancers, but the development of cancer is *not* inevitable. This is usually referred to as *predisposition* or *susceptibility genetic testing*. The description *asymptomatic carrier* is sometimes used for a person who carries a susceptibility or predisposition mutation. Many geneti-

Instructions:
— Evaluation (E) is used to represent clinical and/or test information on the pedigree.
  a. E is to be defined in key/legend.
  b. If more than one evaluation, use subscript (E_1, E_2, E_3) and define in key. May be written
     side by side or below each other depending on available space.
  c. Test results should be put in parentheses or defined in key/legend.
  d. If results of exam/family study/testing not documented or unavailable, may use a question mark (e.g., E?).
— Documented evaluation (*)
  a. Asterisk is placed next to lower right edge of symbol.
  b. Use *only* if examined/evaluated by **you** or *your* research/clinical team or if the outside evaluation has been
     personally reviewed and verified.
— A symbol is shaded only when an individual is clinically symptomatic.
— For linkage studies, haplotype information is written below the individual. The haplotype of interest should
  be on left and appropriately highlighted.
— Repetitive sequences, trinucleotides and expansion numbers are written with affected allele first and
  placed in parentheses.
— If mutation known, identify and place in parentheses.
— Recommended order of information:
  1) age/date of birth or age at death
  2) evaluation information
  3) pedigree number (e.g., I-1, I-2, I-3)

Definition	Symbol	Scenario	Example
1. Documented evaluation (*)		Woman with normal physical exam and negative fragile X chromosome study (normal phenotype and negative test result).	E−
2. Obligate carrier (will **not** manifest disease).		Woman with normal physical exam and premutation for fragile X (normal phenotype and positive test result).	E+(100n/35n)
3. Asymptomatic/presymptomatic carrier (clinically unaffected at this time but could later exhibit symptoms)		Man age 25 with normal physical exam and positive DNA test for Huntington disease (symbol filled in if/when symptoms develop).	25 E+(45n/18n)
4. Uninformative study (u)	E	Man age 25 with normal physical exam and uninformative DNA test for Huntington disease (E_1) and negative brain MRI study (E_2).	25 E_1u(36n/18n) E_2−
5. Affected individual with positive evaluation (E+)	E	Individual with cystic fibrosis and positive mutation study, although only one mutation has currently been identified.	E+(F508) E E+(F508/u)
		18 week male fetus with abnormalities on ultrasound and a trisomy 18 karyotype.	P 18 wk E+(tri 18)

Figure 3.9 How to document results of medical evaluations and genetic testing on a pedigree (including presymptomatic testing and obligate carrier status) (reprinted with permission from Bennett et al., 1995, University of Chicago Press).

cists take exception to the use of the terminology "predictive testing" because no genetic test provides an absolute predictive gaze into a person's medical future.

A person who "carries" a gene mutation but will *not* develop clinical symptoms is referred to as an *obligate carrier* (Bennett et al., 1995). For example, the parents of children affected with a classic autosomal recessive disorder are obligate carriers. A healthy mother of two boys with an X-linked recessive condition (such as Duchenne muscular dystrophy) is an obligate carrier.

Figure 3.9 demonstrates how to document genetic test results, and asymptomatic/presymptomatic and obligate carrier status. Individuals who are obligate carriers are represented on the pedigree with a dot in the middle of the male (square) or female (circle) symbol. Persons who are asymptomatic or presymptomatic carriers are represented with a line down the middle of the pedigree symbol. If the person later develops the disease, the symbol is shaded.

PEDIGREE ETIQUETTE

The Skeletons in the Closet

For many reasons, people tend to keep genetic information private. There is often a sense of stigmatization, even embarrassment, about the "bad blood" or "curse" in the family. An episode from the popular television series *Northern Exposure* described a person with a potential genetic disorder as a "genetic Chernobyl" (Nelkin, 1998). As Francis Galton observed, "Most men and women shrink from having their hereditary worth recorded. There may be family diseases of which they hardly dare to speak, except on rare occasions, and then in whispered hints, or obscure phrases, as though timidity of utterance could hush thoughts . . ." (Resta, 1995). People may also be reluctant to share information because of fear they will be "blamed" for the "family imperfections."

Choose Your Words Wisely

When you take a medical family history, you are inquiring about the very essence of an individual. You are asking not only about the individual's personal health, but also about their intimate relationships and the health of family members (with whom they may have little contact). Before you begin taking a genetic family history, it is helpful to warn the client: "I need to ask you some personal questions about the health of people in your family. Your answers to these questions are an important part of providing you with appropriate medical care."

The clinician should be careful not to perpetuate feelings of guilt and stigmatization. Use words such as "altered" or "changed" to describe genes, instead of "mutated" or "bad." Emphasize to the patient that people have no choice in the genetic conditions that are "passed" in a family; the disease is nobody's fault.

Be sensitive to terms like an "uneventful pregnancy." Although a healthy pregnancy may be uneventful to the clinician, it is very eventful to the proud parents! I often hear clinicians refer to a family history with no apparent genetic problems as a "negative" family history, as compared to a "positive" family history if a genetic condition exists. A "positive" family history is usually very "negative" for the patient (Fisher, 1996)! I usually describe health problems in the family history as being "contributory" or "noncontributory" to the medical problem in question.

Acknowledge Significant Life Events

Common courtesy should be the rule in taking a family history. If a woman tells you that she recently miscarried, or that her mother died of breast cancer a few months ago, it is appropriate to acknowledge this with "I am sorry to hear of your loss" or "This must be a difficult time for you." Conversely, the news of a recent birth, marriage, or desired pregnancy can be greeted with "Congratulations."

Beware the Leading Question

If you say, "So, your brothers and sisters are healthy, right? No problems in your parents?" you will most likely receive a reply of "Un-huh," regardless of whether or not this is a true statement. Instead, try to be specific with your questioning by asking, "Do your brothers and sisters have any health problems?"

Use Common Language

You are more likely to be successful in obtaining an accurate family history if you use terms that are familiar to people. Rather than asking about myopathies in the family, inquire if individuals have muscle weakness, or if anyone uses a cane or a wheelchair?

Be Sensitive to Cultural Issues

If your patient does not speak English, get an interpreter. Do not rely on a family member to provide interpretation. The family member may be tempted to interject his or her opinions, particularly about "family matters," as part of the translation!

Culture consists of shared patterns, knowledge, meaning, and behaviors of a social group (Fisher, 1996). Individuals have different customs and beliefs based on their race, socioeconomic status, sex, religious beliefs, sexual orientation, education, or health status. When taking a family history, it is important to acknowledge belief systems that are different from one's own. For example, a traditional Latino woman may believe that her child's cleft lip and palate are the result of supernatural forces during a lunar eclipse (Cohen et al, 1998). Individuals from a traditional Southeast Asian culture may have strong belief in karma and fate. Persons from certain religious and cultural groups may believe bad thoughts or sins cause a birth defect or genetic disorder (Cohen et al., 1998). References to "bad" things in genetic counseling may disturb the "good aura" of the family or ancestors (Fisher and Lew, 1996).

An individual's belief system is likely to influence the type of health information he or she shares with the health care provider. A vivid example of this is a Hopi woman with severely disabling congenital kyphoscoliosis who was described by her sister as being small and having pain in her legs and back that kept her from her normal activities. The woman was not portrayed as disabled because she had high status in the community due to her ability to make piki, a thin wafer bread (Hauck and Knoki-Wilson, 1996).

Two excellent references on providing health care for diverse population groups are *Cultural and Ethnic Diversity: A Guide for Genetics Professionals*, edited by Nancy Fisher, and *Developing Cross-Cultural Competence: A Guide For Working with Young Children and Their Families,* by Eleanor Lynch and Marci Hanson.

RECORDING A BASIC PEDIGREE: THE QUESTIONS TO ASK

Obtaining an extended medical-family history is really no different from obtaining the medical history from an individual. I usually inform the consultant, "I will now ask you questions about you and your extended family. I am interested in your family members who are both living and dead." Then I ask general questions, reviewing medical systems "from head to toe." If a "positive history" is found, I ask directed questions based on that "system," and the genetic diseases that are associated with it. For additional directed family history questions focused on a positive family history for several common medical conditions (e.g., mental retardation, hearing loss), see Chapter 4.

Medical-Family History Queries by Systems Review

Head, Face, and Neck

Begin by asking, "Does anyone have anything unusual about the way he or she looks?" If yes, have the historian describe the unusual facial features. In particular, inquire about unusual placement or shape of the eyes and ears.

Anyone with an unusually large or small head?

Are there problems with vision, blindness, cataracts, or glaucoma? If so, inquire as to the age the problems began, the severity, and any treatment.

Anyone with unusual eye coloring? For example, eyes that are different colors, or whites of the eyes that are blue?

Do any family members have cleft lip, with or without cleft palate?

Anyone with unusual problems with his or her teeth (e.g., missing, extra, misshapen, fragile, early teeth loss)?

Any problems with hearing or speech?

Anyone with a short or webbed neck?

Anything unusual about the hair (e.g., coarse, fine, early balding, white patch)?

Skeletal System

Is any family member unusually tall or short? (If so, record the heights of the individuals, the parents, and siblings.)

If someone is short, is he or she in proportion or not?

Anyone with curvature of the spine? If so, did this require surgery or bracing?

Anyone with multiple fractures? If yes, inquire as to how many fractures, how the breaks occurred, the bones that were broken, and the age the fractures occurred.

Anyone with an unusual shape to his or her chest?

Anyone with unusually formed bones?

Anyone with unusually long or short fingers or toes? Anyone with extra or missing fingers or toes, or an unusual shape to the hands or feet? Have the historian describe these anomalies.

Anyone with joint problems such that they are unusually stiff or flexible, or dislocate frequently?

Skin

Anyone with unusual lumps, bumps, or birthmarks? If so, have the patient describe them, their location, their coloration, and number. "Were these skin changes ever biopsied or treated?"

Any problems with excessive bruising, or problems with healing or scarring?

Anyone with unusual problems with fingernails or toenails, such as absent nails or growths under the nails?

Respiratory System

Any family members with any lung diseases? If so, were they smokers? Were they treated for the lung condition, and how?

Cardiac System

Anyone with heart disease? If so, at what age, and how were they treated?

Was anyone born with a heart defect? If so, did they have birth defects or mental retardation?

Anyone with heart murmurs?

Anyone with high blood pressure?

Were there any heart surgeries? If so, what was done?

Gastrointestinal System

Anyone with stomach or intestinal tract problems? If so, were they treated for the problem, and how?

Renal System

Anyone with kidney disease? If so, were they treated for the problem, and how? Any problems with alcohol?

Hematologic System

Anyone with bleeding, clotting, or healing problems?
Have any family members been told they are anemic?
Have there been family members who needed transfusions?

Endocrine

Anyone with thyroid problems? Anyone with diabetes? Anyone who is overly heavy or thin?

Immune System

Anyone with frequent infections or hospitalizations, or difficulties healing?

Reproduction

Have any relatives had miscarriages or babies who died, severe pregnancy complications, or infertility?

Neurological/Neuromuscular

Anyone with muscle weakness, or with problems with walking? Do any family members use a cane or wheelchair? If there are muscle problems, inquire as to the age at which the problems began and what type of testing was done, such as a muscle biopsy, nerve conduction velocity, or brain imaging.
Anyone with strokes or seizures? If so, at what age did they begin, and what medications were given?
Anyone with uncontrolled movements, tics, difficulties with coordination, or spasticity? If so, at what age did they begin? Were medications given?
Anyone with slurred speech?

Mental Functioning

Anyone in the family with mental retardation or severe learning problems? Did anyone attend special classes or school, or need help to finish school? If yes, describe the level of functioning and any dysmorphic features. Was the mother taking any drugs, alcohol or medications during the pregnancy; or was she ill?

Are there any family members with problems with thinking or judgment, mental illness, or severe depression? (If so, have the patient describe the relative's symptoms, the age symptoms began, and any known medications.)

General Interview Questions

Occupation   Asking about a patient's occupation helps develop rapport. It also may be a clue to a potential environmental exposure that is contributing to a disease.

Birth Defects   I also ask near the end of the interview if any family members had children with birth defects, particularly of the heart, spine, hands, or feet.

Drug and Alcohol Abuse   Knowing about drug and alcohol abuse in the patient and other family members is important for many reasons. If there are abnormal ultrasound findings in a pregnancy, or a child has birth defects with or without mental retardation, there could be a maternal teratogenic etiology for the problems. The known and suspected human teratogens are list in Table 3.2. Neurological problems can also be related to, or exacerbated by, drug and alcohol use.

There are three specific areas to note when inquiring about possible maternal teratogens:

1. What is the drug or medicine? For medications, ask the patient to bring her prescription to the appointment.
2. When in pregnancy did you take the medication?
3. How much did you take?

When inquiring about a patient's drug and alcohol use, remember that people invariably *underestimate* usage. Do not ask, "Are you a heavy drinker?" Your patient will not want to be judged, and will probably reply "No." Instead ask, "How much alcohol do (did) you use?" or "What drugs do (did) you take?"

Cancer   I usually specifically ask about cancers in the family, because this information may not be volunteered in the medical systems review. Inquire about any family members with cancer, the types of primary cancers, the age of onset, and treatments if known (such as a mastectomy, colectomy, or chemotherapy). Also ask about potential environmental exposures (such as smoking) or occupational exposures. The details of inquiring about specific familial cancer syndromes are outlined in Chapter 5.

TABLE 3.2   Human Teratogens: Proven, Possible, and Unlikely

Known Teratogens

Radiation
  Atomic weapons
  Radioiodine
  Therapeutic radiation
Maternal infections
  Cytomegalovirus (CMV)
  Herpes simplex virus I and II
  Parvovirus B-19
  Rubella virus
  Syphilis
  Toxoplasmosis
  Varicella virus
  Venezuelan equine encephalitis
Maternal and metabolic factors
  Alcoholism
  Early amniocentesis (before day 70
    post-conception)
  Chorionic villus sampling (before
    day 60 post-conception)
  Cretinism, endemic
  Diabetes
  Folic acid deficiency
  Hyperthermia
  Phenylketonuria
  Rheumatic disease
  Sjogren's syndrome
  Virilizing tumors
Drugs and environmental chemicals
  Excessive alcohol
  Aminopterin
  Androgenic hormones
  Busulfan
  Captopril
  Chlorobiphenyls
  Cocaine
  Coumarin anticoagulants
  Cyclophosphamide
  Diethylstilbestrol
  Enalapril
  Etretinate
  Iodides
  Isotretinoin (Accutane®)
  Lithium
  Mercury, organic
  Methotrexate (methylaminopterin)

Methylene blue (via intramniotic injection)
Misoprostol
Methimazole
Penicillamine
Phenytoin (Hydantoin)
Tetracyclines
Thalidomide
Toluene (abuse)
Trimethadione
Valproic acid

Possible Teratogens

  Binge alcohol use
  Carbamazepine
  Cigarette smoking
  Colchicine
  Disulfiram
  Ergotamine
  Fluconazole (high doses)
  Lead
  Primidone
  Quinine (suicidal doses)
  Streptomycin
  Vitamin A (high doses)
  Zinc deficiency

Unlikely Teratogens

  Agent Orange
  Anesthetics
  Aspartame
  Aspirin[a]
  Bendectin
  Hydroxyprogesterone
  LSD
  Marijuana
  Medroxyprogesterone
  Metronidazole
  Oral contraceptives
  Progesterone
  Rubella vaccine
  Spermicides
  Video display terminals and
    electromagnetic waves
  Ultrasound

[a]Aspirin use may increase cerebral hemorrhage during delivery if used in the second half of pregnancy.
Source: Adapted from Cohen, 1997; Shepard, 1996.

Ethnicity   Inquiring about ethnicity is one of the last questions to ask when taking a pedigree. Certain genetic conditions, particularly autosomal recessive disorders, are more common in certain ethnic groups (see Table 3.3 and Chapter 2). For some genetic disorders, the sensitivity of DNA testing depends on the person's ethnicity. The ethnicity should be recorded for all four of the grandparents of the consultand. Usually this information is placed at the top of the pedigree, at the head of each lineage. If ethnicity is unknown, you can draw a question mark or write "unknown" at the top of the lineage.

Patients may wonder why you are inquiring about their ethnic background. They may fear that you have singled out their ethnic group for genetic screening or testing. I usually say, "Information about the origins of your ancestors can help us offer you the most appropriate genetic information and testing. Do you know your country of origin, where your ancestors were originally from?" You may get a reply of "South Dakota or Nebraska", to which I reply, "Can you be more specific? For instance, were your ancestors Black, Spanish, Native American, or European?." If someone is Native American, it is helpful to ask the tribal background. Likewise, knowing the village name from small countries is useful.

Because more and more genetic tests are becoming available to people of Ashke-

Table 3.3   Genetic Disorders That Have a High Incidence in Certain Ethnic Groups

Population Group	Condition	Inheritance Pattern[a]	Approximate Prevalence
African (Central)	Sickle cell anemia	AR	1/50
Ashkenazi Jewish	Gaucher type I disease	AR	1/1000
	Cystic fibrosis	AR	1/3300
	Tay–Sachs disease	AR	1/3600
	Familial dysautonomia	AR	1/3700
	Canavan disease	AR	1/6400
Caucasian	Phenyketonuria (PKU)	AR	1/20,000
	Cystic fibrosis	AR	1/3300
French Canadian (Saguenay-Lac Saint-Jean)	Tyrosinemia	AR	5.4/10,000
South African (white)	Porphyria variegata	AD	3/1000
Yupik Eskimo	Congenital adrenal hyperplasia	AR	1/500
Turkish	PKU	AR	3.8/10,000
Yemenite Jewish	PKU	AR	1.9/10,000
Ojibway Indian (Canada)	Glutaric aciduria I	AR	1/2000
Hopi Native American	Oculoctaneous albinism II	AR	1/227
Pueblo Native American	Cystic fibrosis	AR	1/3970
Zuni Native American	Cystic fibrosis	AR	1/1580
Swedish	Glutaric aciduria I	AR	3.3/100,000
Mennonite (Pennsylvania)	Maple syrup urine disease	AR	56.8/10,000
Amish (Eastern Pennsylvania)	Ellis van Creveld	AR	1/700
	Glutaric aciduria I	AR	1/400
Finnish	Congenital nephrotic syndrome	AR	1/8000

[a]AR—autosomal recessive, AD—autosomal dominant.
Sources: Clarke, 1996; NIH Consensus Statement, 1997; OMIM, 1998; Scriver et al., 1995.

nazi Jewish heritage, I specifically ask, "Is anyone in your family of Jewish heritage?"

Never assume ethnicity by dress, skin color, or language. I learned this the hard way once when I requested a Spanish interpreter for a non-English speaking client. When a Japanese gentleman arrived from interpreter services, I said, "Oh, you must be in the wrong clinic." He politely informed me that I was the one who was misinformed.

It's All Relative: Consanguinity

One of the final pedigree history questions is: "Has anyone in your family ever had a child with a relative? For example, were your parents or grandparents related as cousins?" Often you are greeted with a nervous laugh, and an answer of "not that we know of." In the United States, people are very sensitive to questions about unions between relatives. Marriage between first cousins is legal in about half of the states in America. In some parts of the world, particularly the Middle East, close to half the population is married to a cousin or more distant relative.

People are often confused by the terms describing kinship. For example, a second cousin is commonly confused with a first cousin once removed (Fig. 3.10). It is important to work "back" through the family history to document exactly how the couple is related. For example, the clinician might say, "Let me see if I have this straight, your father and your wife's mother are brother and sister, therefore you are first cousins." If the degree of relationship is not implicit from the pedigree, it should be stated above the relationship line, as shown in the pedigree of the prestigious Darwin and Wedgwood families (Fig. 3.11).

Individuals from different branches of the family, with the same last name, may

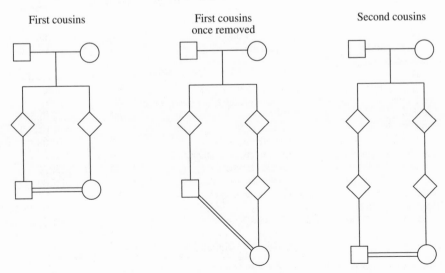

First cousins

First cousins
once removed

Second cousins

Figure 3.10 Symbolization of first cousins, first cousins once removed, and second cousins.

be distantly related. Ancestors from the same small tribes or villages may also be consanguineous.

Documenting that you have inquired about consanguinity should be noted on every pedigree. The information "consanguinity denied," or "consanguinity as shown" can be incorporated into the key, or written near the top of the pedigree.

The Closing Questions

Before I finish the interview, I always end with these questions: "Aside from the information that you have given me, is there anything that people say 'runs' in your family? Do you have any other questions about something that you are concerned may be genetic or inherited in your family? Is there anything that I have not asked you about, that you feel is important for me to know?" Patients always seem to save their burning questions for the last few minutes of their appointment! Perhaps it takes them some time to warm up to the interview. Maybe they are embarrassed about something in their family history. Or possibly nervousness just causes temporary memory loss. Regardless of the reason, always provide the consultand with a final opportunity to think about additional concerns in his or her medical–family history.

The Family Photo Album

If a person in the family is described as having unusual facial or other physical features, have your patient raid the family photo album. Pictures from a wedding or family reunion are an easy way to see if people resemble each other. Such pictures are also a way to determine if an individual is unusually tall or short for the family. Summer pictures of a beach outing show more "flesh," if you are trying to investigate unusual skeletal features or skin findings. Looking at chronological pictures of the same individual over a several year period can be useful; some syndromes may be difficult to identify in childhood, or may be less obvious in an adult than in a child.

WHAT'S REMARKABLE ABOUT AN UNREMARKABLE FAMILY HISTORY?

Many times when you take a family history, there are no obvious genetic diseases or familial aggregation of disease. Table 3.4 reviews some common reasons that a family history of a genetic condition is missed. Clinicians often note in the medical record that the family history is "negative" or the person has "no family history." I prefer stating the family history is unremarkable or noncontributory. The word "negative" may be misconstrued as a value judgment. All humans have a family history, though the medical–family history may not affect the current indication for seeing a health professional.

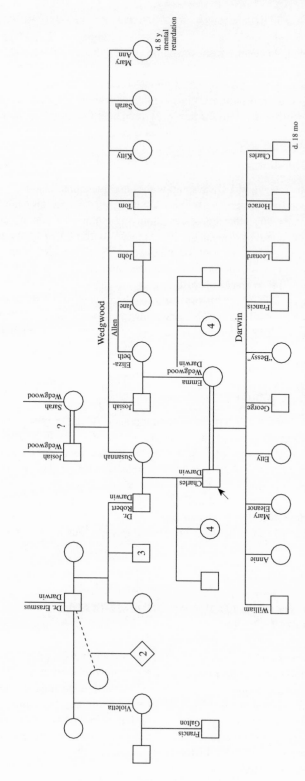

Figure 3.11 A pedigree of first cousins, Charles Darwin and his wife Emma Wedgwood Darwin. Their mutual grandparents, Josiah and Sarah Wedgwood, were also related as cousins.

TABLE 3.4   Possible Explanations for a Seemingly Unremarkable Family History

Individual has a new mutation (dominant, mitochondrial)
New X-linked mutation (in a male)
Affected person is not the natural child of parent(s) (e.g., nonpaternity, adoption, artificial insemination by donor semen)
Sex-limited inheritance
Seemingly unaffected parent actually has subtle expression of disease/syndrome (always examine the parents!)
Delayed age of onset of symptoms
Reduced penetrance
Small family size
Failure of the clinician to take a three-generation pedigree
Lack of knowledge of person giving history to clinician
Intentional withholding of information by historian (i.e., person may feel guilty or embarrassed, or fear discrimination)

WHEN IS A GENETIC FAMILY HISTORY SIGNIFICANT?

This is a tough question to answer. My feeling is that a significant family history is one that the patient is concerned about, or one that the patient *should* be concerned about. A 22-year-old woman with an abnormal ultrasound finding at 16 weeks may have a strong family history of breast and ovarian cancer, but a desire for information about inherited cancer susceptibility testing is probably the farthest thing from her mind at that moment. Instead, delving further into this information at a future visit is warranted, and might be communicated to the woman in a follow-up letter.

THE ULTIMATE PEDIGREE CHALLENGE

The following fictitious family history is provided for you to practice drawing each standardized pedigree symbol. This teaching scenario is republished with permission from the American Journal of Human Genetics (Bennett et al., 1995). The "answer" is in Appendix A.1.

The consultand, Mrs. Feene O'Type, presents to your office with a pregnancy at 16 wk gestation. She has questions about risks to her fetus because of her age. She is 35 years old and her husband, Gene O'Type, is 36 years old. Mrs. O'Type had one prior pregnancy, an elective termination (TOP) at 18 wk, of a female fetus with trisomy 21.

Mrs. O'Type's Family History

- Mrs. O'Type had three prior pregnancies with her first husband. The first pregnancy was a TOP, the second a spontaneous abortion (SAB) of a female fetus at 19 wk gestation, and the third a healthy 10-year-old son who was subsequently adopted by her 33-year-old sister, Stacy.

- Stacy had three pregnancies, two SABs (the second a male fetus at 20 wk with a neural tube defect and a karyotype of trisomy 18) and a stillborn female at 32 wk.

- Mrs. O'Type has a 31-year-old brother, Sam, who is affected with cystic fibrosis (CF) and is infertile.

- Her youngest brother, Donald, age 29 years, is healthy and married. By means of gametes from Donald and his wife, an unrelated surrogate mother has been successfully impregnated.

- Mrs. O'Type's father died at age 72 years and her mother at age 70 years, both from "natural causes." Mrs. O'Type's mother had five healthy full sibs, who themselves had many healthy children.

Mr. O'Type's Family History

- Mr. O'Type has two siblings, a monozygotic twin brother, Cary, whose wife is 6 wk pregnant by donor insemination (donor's history unknown), and a 32-year old sister, Sterrie.

- Sterrie is married to Proto, her first cousin (Sterrie's father's sister's son), who has red/green color blindness. She is carrying a pregnancy conceived from Proto's sperm, and ovum from an unknown donor. Sterrie and Proto also have an adopted son.

- The family history of Sterrie's mother, who has Huntington disease (HD), is unknown.

- Mr. Gene O'Type's father has a set of twin brothers, zygosity unknown, and another brother and sister (Proto's mother), who are also twins.

REFERENCES

Bennett RL, Steinhaus KA, Uhrich SB, et al. (1995). Recommendations for standardized human pedigree nomenclature. Am J Hum Genet 56:745–752.

Brinkman RR, Mezei MM, Theilmann J, Almqvuist E, Hayden MR (1997). The likelihood of being affected with Huntington disease by a particular age, for a specific CAG size. Am J Hum Genet 60:1202–1210.

Cohen MM (1997). *The Child with Multiple Birth Defects,* 2nd ed. New York: Oxford University Press.

Cohen LH, Fine BA, Pergament (1998). An assessment of ethnocultural beliefs regarding the causes of birth defects and genetic disorders. J Genet Couns 7:15–29.

Fisher NL (ed) (1996). *Cultural and Ethnic Diversity. A Guide for Genetics Professionals.* Baltimore: Johns Hopkins University Press.

Fisher NL, Lew L (1996). Culture of the countries of Southeast Asia. In Fisher NF (ed), *Cultural and Ethnic Diversity, A Guide for Genetics Professionals.* Baltimore: Johns Hopkins University Press, pp. 113–128.

Hauck L, Knoki-Wilson UM (1996). Culture of Native Americans of the Southwest. In Fisher NF (ed), *Cultural and Ethnic Diversity, A Guide for Genetics Professionals*. Baltimore: Johns Hopkins University Press, pp. 60–85.

Lynch EW, Hanson MJ (1992). *Developing Cross-Cultural Competence. A Guide for Working with Young Children and Their Families*. Baltimore: Paul H. Brookes Publishing Co.

Marazita ML (1995). Defining "proband." Am J Hum Genet 57:981–82.

Nelkin D (1998). Cancer genetics and public expectations. In Foulkes WD, Hodgson SV (eds), *Inherited Susceptibility to Cancer: Clinical, Predictive and Ethical Perspectives*. Cambridge: Cambridge University Press, p. 55.

NIH Consensus Statement (1997 Apr 14–16). Genetic Testing for Cystic Fibrosis. 15(4):1–37.

Online Mendelian Inheritance in Man, OMIM™. Center for Medical Genetics, Johns Hopkins University (Baltimore, MD), 1997. Accessed June 19, 1998. World Wide Web URL: http://www.ncbi.nlm.nih.gov/omim/

Resta RG (1993). The crane's foot: the rise of the pedigree in human genetics. J Genet Couns 2(4):235–260.

Resta RG (1995). Whispered hints. Am J Med Genet 59:131–133.

Scriver CR, Beaudet AL, Sly WS, Valle D (eds) (1995). *The Metabolic and Molecular Bases of Inherited Disease*, 7th ed. New York: McGraw-Hill.

Shepard TH (1996). *Catalog of Teratogenic Agents*, 8th ed. Baltimore: The Johns Hopkins University Press.

4

Directed Medical-Genetic Family History Queries: Separating the Trees from the Forest

Genetic cases sometimes hide in a chiaroscuro of common disease patterns . . .
Generalists will usher in the millennium with genetic tests for cancer predisposition and
Alzheimer disease. Genetic risk is a new axis of disease, requiring critical test
interpretation, skillful counseling, and dedicated follow-up of families . . . Do today's
peculiarities in medical genetics presage tomorrow's primary care?
*—**Wendy S. Rubinstein (1997)***

4.1 THE APPROACH: LOOK FOR THE RARE BUT REMEMBER THE ORDINARY

Patients and family members often inquire about the heritability of common medical conditions. This chapter provides suggestions for directed family history questions related to many of the everyday medical diseases encountered in the "typical" family history. By supplementing general family history screening questions (as reviewed in Chapter 3) with a more targeted query, the clinician can probe deeper into the medical-family history and identify individuals who may benefit from a more extensive genetic evaluation and genetic counseling. To borrow from a common proverb, these screening questions are a method to distinguish the unusual trees from the vast forest. As with any "field guide," often it is best to look to the experts for final identification. Resources for making a patient referral for genetic services can be found in Chapter 11. Some of the "red flags" in a medical-family history that suggest a genetic etiology of disease are reviewed in Table 4.1.

Instead of discussing the potential genetic disorders associated with every common medical condition, I shall focus on a selection of medical-family history signposts representative of medical conditions with a potential hereditary etiology. For example, leukemia, although a rare complication of Down syndrome, is not a useful "signpost" for recognizing this condition because an infant with Down syndrome is more readily diagnosed by other "signposts." In contrast, leukemia is a common cancer in children and adults in the familial cancer syndrome Li–Fraumeni (see Chapter 5). In this instance, knowing more about the family history can aid the clinician in deciding on genetic testing and health management strategies for relevant family members. The patient's answers to such targeted queries can be transposed into a medical pedigree and used as an investigative map to assist with diagnosis and risk appraisal.

In this chapter I provide suggestions for medical-family history queries for the following broad categories of disease: birth anomalies (Section 4.2), hearing loss (Section 4.3), visual impairment (Section 4.4), mental retardation (Section 4.5), autism (Section 4.6), neurological conditions (Section 4.7), seizures (Section 4.8), dementia (Section 4.9), mental illness (Section 4.10), cardiac disease (Section 4.11), chronic respiratory disease (Section 4.12), renal disorders (Section 4.13), short stature (Section 4.14), diabetes (Section 4.15), reproductive loss and infertility (Section 4.16), and sudden infant death (Section 4.17). Family history markers for identifying individuals with an inherited susceptibility to cancer are discussed in Chapter 5. The decision to include these general groupings of disease in this chapter is based on my experience with some of the questions people have asked me most frequently about disorders in their family.

I do not provide information on the diagnostic tests and the clinical signs and symptoms of the many genetic disorders mentioned in this chapter, nor do I discuss the essential genetic counseling and psychosocial issues for each condition. I do mention several situations where obtaining a medical-family history poses special challenges (such as obtaining a history from a person with profound hearing loss, or from an individual with severe learning disabilities). There are many excellent and comprehensive tomes delving into the medical and psychosocial intricacies of hereditary disease (see Appendix A.5: The Genetics Library).

The key to teasing out potential genetic variables in a patient's family history is to look for unusual and infrequent features against a background of common diseases and normal physical variation. Male infertility is common, but a man with infertility, small testes (hypogonadism), and absence of the sense of smell (anosmia), may have a rare inherited condition called Kallman syndrome. Diabetes mellitus is a common chronic disorder, but a person with diabetes, seizures, hearing loss, and an unsteady gait may have a mitochondrial myopathy.

As clinicians, when we recognize a set of "peculiarities" as a "genetic case" (paraphrasing Dr. Rubinstein in the introductory quote to this chapter), it is natural to swell with a peacock's pride at our diagnostic prowess. It is easy for us to lose sight of the person behind the "peculiar" signs and symptoms. Observes a parent of

TABLE 4.1   The Red Flags in a Medical-Family History Suggestive of a Genetic Condition or an Inherited Susceptibility to a Common Disease

- Multiple closely related individuals affected with the same condition, particularly if the condition is rare
- Common disorders with earlier age of onset than typical (especially if onset is early in multiple family members). For example:
  Breast cancer < age 45–50 years (premenopausal)
  Colon cancer < age 45–50 years
  Prostate cancer < age 50–60 years
  Vision loss < age 55 years
  Hearing loss < age 50–60 years
  Dementia < age 60 years
  Heart disease < age 40–50 years
- Bilateral disease in paired organs (e.g., eyes, kidneys, lungs, breasts)
- Sudden cardiac death in a person who seemed healthy
- Individual or couple with three or more pregnancy losses (e.g., miscarriages, stillbirths)
- Medical problems in the offspring of parents who are consanguineous (first cousins or more closely related)

A person with:
- Two or more medical conditions (e.g., hearing loss and renal disease, diabetes and muscle disease)
- A medical condition and dysmorphic features
- Developmental delay with dysmorphic features and/or physical birth anomalies
- Developmental delay associated with other medical conditions
- Progressive mental retardation, loss of developmental milestones
- Progressive behavioral problems
- Unexplained hypotonia
- A movement disorder
- Unexplained seizures
- Unexplained ataxia
- Two or more major birth anomalies (see Table 4.3)
- Three or more minor birth anomalies (see Table 4.3)
- One major birth defect with two minor anomalies
- A cleft palate, or cleft lip with or without cleft palate
- Unusual birthmarks (particularly if associated with seizures, learning disabilities, or dysmorphic features)
- Hair anomalies (hirsute, brittle, coarse, kinky, sparse or absent)
- Congenital or juvenile deafness
- Congenital or juvenile blindness
- Cataracts at a young age
- Primary amenorrhea
- Ambiguous genitalia
- Proportionate short stature with dysmorphic features and/or delayed or arrested puberty
- Disproportionate short stature
- Premature ovarian failure
- Proportionate short stature and primary amenorrhea
- Males with hypogonadism and/or significant gynecomastia
- Congenital absence of the vas deferens
- Oligozoospermia/azoospermia

A fetus with:
- a major structural anomaly
- significant growth retardation
- or multiple minor anomalies

a child with a "rare" condition, "A condition is only rare when it happens in some-one else's family." Carolyn, a woman with multiple birth anomalies who wept after her astute genetic counselor remarked on her beautiful feet, touchingly recalls the profound impact of constantly having clinicians point only to her peculiarities:

> Over the years I've seen a lot of doctors. Every one of them has described in excruciating detail what was wrong with me. After a while, I began to feel like no part of me was normal. But deep down inside, I always felt I had beautiful feet. I knew my arm was misshapen, and I knew I didn't have periods like oth-er women, and even my kidneys, which worked fine and people couldn't see, were abnormal. But my feet . . . from the knees down, I thought I looked like every woman. As odd as it sounds, having that little bit of security has helped me get through some tough days. Then, 5 years ago, a doctor casually men-tioned that my feet look abnormal. His words were not said cruelly, but they crushed me. The last part of me which I had clung to as normal had been de-stroyed by what that doctor said. When you just told me now that my feet look normal, it brought back the memory of that day when my whole self-image collapsed (Resta, 1997).

Behind each "genetic case" is a person and family with normal dreams, thoughts, and feelings.

4.2 PHYSICAL BIRTH ANOMALIES AND VARIANTS

A family history of birth defects is usually a major concern to a couple making re-productive choices. It is not unusual to encounter a family history of a significant birth defect; an estimated 3% of newborns have one or more major physical anom-alies. As many as 1/3 of congenital anomalies are characterized as being genetic in origin. Known environmental teratogens (see Table 3.2) are surprisingly few, and they are implicated as causal factors in approximately 1/400 birth anomalies (Win-ter et al., 1988). The etiology of as many as half of all birth defects is unknown (Kalter and Warkany, 1983).

Physical anomalies that are recognized at birth or in infancy are categorized as major or minor. Major anomalies (such as an omphalocele, most congenital heart defects, or a facial cleft) are of medical and/or cosmetic significance. Table 4.2 gives examples of major congenital anomalies. Minor malformations (usually in-volving the face, ears, hands, and feet) affect somewhere between 4 and 15% of the population. (Cohen et al., 1997; Cohen, 1997; Robinson and Linden, 1993). Minor anomalies do not have substantial medical or cosmetic consequences. A minor anomaly seen without other physical differences may represent the spectrum of nor-mal variation, and it may be inherited. Learning disabilities and mental retardation are often associated with syndromes involving birth anomalies. Before a minor vari-ation is considered significant, the parents (and other family members) should be examined to see if the characteristic is simply a normal familial variant. For exam-ple, it is common for syndactyly of the second and third toes to be familial.

TABLE 4.2   Examples of Major Congenital Anomalies[a]

Brain malformations	Neural tube defects (NTD)
Holoprosencephaly	Anencephaly
Microcephaly	Spina bifida
Cleft lip with or without cleft palate (CL/P)	Encephalocele
Cleft palate	Myelomeningocele
Esophageal atresia	Omphalocele
Microtia, or anotia	Gastroschisis
Microphthalmos, or anophthalmos	Diaphragmatic hernia
Congenital heart defects	Duodenal atresia
Atrial septal defect (ASD)	Imperforate anus (anal atresia)
Coarctation of the aorta	Polydactyly
Double-outlet right ventricle	Absence of thumb or other digits
Ebstein anomaly	Arthrogryposis
Ectopia cordis	Limb anomalies
Endocardial cushion defect	Absence (agenesis) of any organ
Hypoplastic left-heart syndrome (HLHS)	Renal agenesis
Tetralogy of Fallot	Gonadal agenesis
Transposition of the great arteries (TGA)	
Ventricular septal defect (VSD)	

[a]All terms are defined in the Glossary.

The identification of minor birth anomalies and differences is an essential component of syndrome recognition (a syndrome is a combination of causally related physical variants). A simian crease (a single line across the palm versus the more usual transverse parallel lines) is a normal finding in 3% of the general population but it is a clinical finding in almost half of all neonates with Down syndrome (Jones, 1997). A person who has three minor birth anomalies, or a major anomaly with two anomalies, is likely to have a syndrome. An individual with three or more minor anomalies should also be evaluated for underlying major malformations (such as a heart defect) (Cohen et al., 1997). Table 4.3 includes examples of minor physical differences detectable at birth or shortly thereafter that may be seen in isolation or as part of a syndrome.

Examining the parents of a child with one or more congenital anomalies is useful for syndrome diagnosis and for determining recurrence risks and prognosis. A child's unusually formed ears may be evident in a parent as a normal familial characteristic. Alternatively, the parent's remarkably shaped ears can be minor manifestations of a variably expressed autosomal dominant syndrome with a more severe presentation evidenced in the child. If both parents of a child with a major birth anomaly have normal physical examinations, it is more reassuring to quote the chances of recurrence from an empirical risk table than if the child is evaluated in isolation from the parents. Comparing photographs of the child, parents, and other family members is an inexpensive and important method for distinguishing normal variation from subtle syndromic expression of a familial characteristic.

Most isolated birth anomalies (major and minor) have a polygenic/multifactorial etiology (see Chapter 2). The parents of a child with an isolated congenital malformation usually have a relatively low recurrence risk (in the range of 3–10%). The

TABLE 4.3 Examples of Minor Physical Differences That can be within Normal Variation or a Feature of a Syndrome (Inherited or Environmental)

Variant Physical Feature	Representative Syndromes[a]
Hair	
Low posterior hairline	Turner s. (CH),[b] Noonan s. (AD)[b]
Upward sweep of hair ("cowlick")	May reflect defective brain (frontal lobe) development and primary microcephaly, and is associated with several syndromes
"Widow's peak"	May be associated with ocular hypertelorism, examples: Aarskog s. (AD, XL),[b] Opitz s. (hypertelorism–hypospadias s.) (AD, XL), Smith–Lemli Opitz s. (AR),[b] Waardenburg s. I and II (AD)
White streak (forelock) of hair	Waardenburg s. I and II (AD)
Synophrys	Sanfillipo s., (AR),[b] deLange s. (IM),[b] fetal trimethadione s. (T)[b]
Hirsutism	Fetal alcohol s. (T),[b] fetal hydantoin s. (T),[b] fetal trimethadione (T),[b] deLange s. (IM),[b] mucopolysaccharidoses (AR, XL)[b]
Sparse, fine hair	Hypohidrotic ectodermal dysplasia (XL)
Ears	
Simple	Fetal alcohol s. (T),[b] fetal hydantoin s. (T)[b]
Protruberant ears	Fragile X s. (XL)[b]
Ear tags	Mandibulofacial dysostosis (Treacher–Collins s.) (AD), OAV (AD)
Ear pits	Branchio-oto-renal s. (AD) (pre-auricular pits)
Microtia	Mandibulofacial dysostosis (Treacher–Collins s.) (AD), OAV (AD)
Creases in ear lobe	Beckwith–Wiedemann s. (IM), familial hyperlipidemia (AD)
Eyes	
Iris coloboma[c]	Several chromosome anomalies, CHARGE association
Blue or gray sclerae	Normal in newborns; osteogenesis imperfecta (AD)
Heterochromia	Waardenburg s. I and II (AD)
Brushfield spots	Seen in 20% of normal newborns, Down s. (CH)[b]
Epicanthal folds	Normal finding in infancy; Down s. (CH)[b] and several other chromosome anomalies, Opitz s. (AD, XL), fetal hydantoin s. (T)[b]
Ptosis	Aarskog s. (AD, XL),[b] myotonic dystrophy (AD),[b] Noonan s. (AD), Smith–Lemli–Opitz s., (AR),[b] fetal hydantoin s. (T)[b]
Hypertelorism	Craniosynostosis syndromes many of which are AD (e.g., Crouzon s., Apert s., Pfeiffer s.), multiple chromosomal syndromes, Noonan s. (AD),[b] Aarskog s. (AD, XL), fetal hydantoin s. (T),[b] oto-palato-digital types I and II, (XL), nevoid basal cell carcinoma s. (NBCCS) (AD), Robinow s. (AD, AR)
Dystopia canthorum	Waardenburg s. I (AD)
Hypotelorism	Trisomy 13 (CH),[b] syndromes with holoprosencephaly
Downward slanting palpebral fissures	Aarskog s. (AD, XL),[b] Opitz s. (AD), Coffin–Lowry s. (XL),[b] Rubenstein–Taybi s.(CH-del)[b]

(continued)

TABLE 4.3 *(continued)*

Variant Physical Feature	Representative Syndromes[a]
Short palpebral fissures	Fetal alcohol s. (T),[b] Dubowitz s. (AR),[b] velocardiofacial s. (AD, CH–del)[b]
Long palpebral fissures	Kabuki s. (?)[b]
Nose	
Prominent, bulbous nose	Velocardiofacial s. (AD, CH–del),[b] TRPS-I (AD),[b] TRPS-II (CH-del),[b] Rubenstein–Taybi s. (CH-del)[b]
Broad nasal bridge	Aarskog s. (AD, XL),[b] Coffin–Lowry s. (XL),[b] Simpson–Golabi–Behmel s. (XL),[b] TRPS I (AD),[b] TRPS-II (CH-del),[b] fetal hydantoin s. (T),[b] nevoid basal cell carcinoma s. (AD), Waardenburg s. I and II (AD)
Philtrum	
Long/flat	Fetal alcohol s. (T),[b] fetal valproate s. (T),[b] de Lange s. (IM)[b], Williams s. (CH-del),[b] TRPS-I (AD),[b] TRPS-II (CH-del),[b] Robinow s. (AD, AR)
Oral region	
Micrognathia	Associated with close to 100 syndromes, many of which are chromosomal or teratogenic. Also seen as a deformation from uterine constriction
Enamel hypoplasia	Osteogenesis imperfecta I (AD)
Wide spaced teeth	Angelman s. (IM),[b] Coffin–Lowry s. (XL)[b]
Peg-shaped teeth	Incontinentia pigmenti[b] (XL-lethal in males)
Conical teeth	Hypohidrotic ectodermal dysplasia (AD), Ellis–van Creveld s./chondroectodermal dysplasia (AR)
Lip pits (pits in lower lip)	Van der Woude s. (AD)
Lip pigmentation	Peutz–Jeghers s. (AD)
Neck	
Webbed neck	Turner s. (CH),[b] Noonan s. (AD)[b]
Hands and feet	
Polydactyly[c] (postaxial)	Trisomy 13 (CH),[b] chondroectodermal dysplasia/Ellis–van Creveld s. (AR), orofacial digital s. (multiple types) (XL, AD, AR),[b] Smith–Lemli–Opitz s. (AR),[b] Simpson–Golabai–Behmel s. (XL),[b] can be inherited as an AD sydrome (particularly in African Americans) with no other anomalies
Polydactyly[c] (preaxial)	Carpenter s. (AR)[b]
Brachydactyly[c]	Can be an AD syndrome with no other anomalies, associated with several multiple congenital anomaly syndromes, fetal aminopterin/methotrexate s. (T)
Metacarpal hypoplasia (short 3rd, 4th, and/or 5th fingers)	Albright hereditary osteodystrophy (AD), nevoid basal cell carcinoma s. (Gorlin s.) (AD), TRPS-1 (AD),[b] TRPS-II (CH-del)[b]
Digitial asymmetry	Oro-facial-digital s. (multiple types) (AD, AR, XL)[b]
Clinodactyly	Down s. and other chromosome anomalies, TRPS-I (AD),[b] TRPS-II (CH-del)[b]
Tapered fingers	Velocardiofacial syndrome (AD, CH–del),[b] Coffin–Lowry s. (XL)[b]
Arachnodactyly	Marfan s. (AD), homocystinuria (AR)[b]
Single palmar (simian) crease	Down s. (CH),[b] Trisomy 13 (CH),[b] Seckel s. (AR),[b] Aarskog s. (AD, XL),[b] Smith–Lemli–Opitz s. (AR),[b] Simpson–Golabi–Behmel s. (XL),[b] deLange s. (IM),[b] fetal trimethadione s. (T)[b]

(continued)

TABLE 4.3   *(continued)*

Variant Physical Feature	Representative Syndromes[a]
Hyperconvex nails	Fetal valproate s. (T),[b] trisomy 13 (CH)[b]
Nail hypoplasia	Williams s. (CH-del),[b] chondroectodermal dysplasia/Ellis–van Creveld s. (AR), Simpson–Golabi–Behmel s. (XL),[b] fetal alcohol s. (T),[b] fetal hydantoin s. (T),[b] fetal coumarin anticoagulants (T),[b] fetal valproate s. (T)[b]
Broad thumbs/toes	Rubenstein–Taybi s. (CH-del),[b] Pfeiffer s. (AD), oto-palato-digital s. I & II (XL),[b] Aarskog s. (AD, XL)[b]
Syndactyly (mild)	Smith–Lemli–Opitz s. (AR),[b] deLange s. (CH-del),[b] oro-facial-digital s. (multiple types) (AR, AD, XL),[b] Pfeiffer s. (AD), Simpson–Golabi–Behmel s. (XL),[b] Aarskog s. (AD, XL),[b] fetal alcohol s. (T)[b]
Gap between big toe (hallux) and 2nd toe	Down s. (CH)[b]
Chest	
Wide spaced nipples	Turner s. (CH),[b] trisomy 18 (CH),[b] TRSP-II (CH-del),[b] fetal hydantoin s. (T)
Supernumerary nipples (accessory or extra)	fetal valproate s. (T),[b] Bannayan–Zonana s. (AD),[b] Simpson–Golabi–Behmel s. (XL),[b] tetrasomy 12p (Pallister–Killian s.) (CH-mosaic),[b] TRPS-II (CH-del)[b]
Skin	
Areas of skin hypopigmentation	Tuberous sclerosis 1 and 2 (ash leaf) (AR),[b] Waardenburg s. (AD)
Café au lait spots	Neurofibromatosis (AD)
Abdominal	
Umbilical hernia[c]	Hurler s. (AR),[b] Beckwith–Wiedemann (AD, IM), trisomy 13 (CH),[b] trisomy 18 (CH),[b] Simpson–Golabi–Behmel s. (XL),[b] velocardiofacial s. (AD, CH–del)[b]
Genitalia	
Shawl scrotum	Aarskog s. (AD, XL)[b]
Hypoplastic labia	Prader–Willi s. (IM),[b] Robinow syndrome (AD, AR)
Small penis	Bardet–Biedel s. (AR),[b] chondroectodermal dysplasia/Ellis–van Creveld s. (AR), Robinow s. (AD, AR), Smith–Lemli–Opitz s. (AR),[b] Prader–Willi s. (IM),[b] Noonan s. (AD)[b]
Hypospadias[c]	Smith–Lemli–Opitz s. (AR),[b] Opitz s. (XL, AD), fetal trimethadione s. (T),[b] deLange s. (IM)[b]
Skeletal	
Cubitis valgus	Aarskog s. (AD, XL),[b] Noonan s. (AD),[b] Turner s. (CH)[b]
Pectus excavatum[c]	Marfan s. (AD), homocystinuria (AR),[b] Aarskog s. (XL),[b] Coffin–Lowry s. (XL),[b] oto-palato-digital s. I and II (XL),[b] Simpson–Golabi–Behmel s. (XL)[b]
Pectus carinatum[c]	Marfan s. (AD), homocystinuria (AR),[b] Coffin–Lowry s. (XL),[b] Robinow s. (AD, AR)

[a]Abbreviations: s. = syndrome; TRPS-1 = trichorhinophalangeal s. type I; TRPS-2 = trichorhinophalangeal s. type II (Langer–Gideon s.); OAV = oculo-auriculo-vertebral spectrum (hemifacial microsomia or Goldenhar syndrome); CH = chromosomal; CH-del = chromosomal deletion; AD = autosomal dominant; AR = autosomal recessive; XL = X-linked; IM = imprinting; T = teratogen; ? = unknown etiology.
[b]Syndrome frequently associated with learning disabilities or mental retardation.
[c]Can be major congenital anomaly.
Sources: Cohen, 1997; Gorlin et al., 1995; Jones, 1997; OMIM, 1998; Sanders, 1996; Sybert, 1997; Tewfik et al., 1997.

risk of recurrence rises if there is another affected child in the family. Of course, if a parent has more than one child with the same congenital anomaly, or if there is a family history of similar birth anomalies, a single gene etiology should be investigated. *This includes examining the parents for physical signs of subtle expression of the condition.* Parental consanguinity is another clue suggesting single gene causation.

Some congenital anomalies are more common in certain ethnic groups. In the United States, cleft lip and palate are more common in people of Asian and Native American descent (~15/10,000 births) than in African Americans (8/10,000 births) (Khoury et al., 1997). Postaxial polydactyly occurs in approximately 1/500 African Americans, and is often inherited in an autosomal dominant pattern within this population group. In providing risk assessment, such ethnic variables are important to consider.

Multiple birth defects (major and minor) are often associated with chromosome anomalies (see Chapter 2). Thus it is important to inquire about a family history of miscarriages, infertility, mental retardation, and other birth defects. Birth defect(s) associated with other features suggest a single gene disorder. Exposure to certain prescription drugs and alcohol during critical periods in embryonic development is associated with various birth defects. Remember to explore the mother's history of alcohol and street and prescription drug use during the pregnancy. Several infectious agents are teratogenic during pregnancy. Table 3.2 reviews known and potential fetal teratogens. When inquiring about a potential teratogenic agent, remember to document when in pregnancy the agent was given (or when an infection occurred), as well as the dosage or amounts of drug taken (see Chapter 3).

Birth defects are divided into three general classifications: *malformations, deformations,* and *disruptions* (Cohen, 1997; Jones, 1997). The distinction between these categories may assist the clinician in determining prognosis, recurrence risk, and appropriate therapeutic interventions.

Malformations are defects in an organ, or part of an organ, resulting from an intrinsically abnormal developmental process. Examples of malformations include syndactyly (webbing of the fingers or toes), polydactyly (extra fingers or toes), congenital heart defects, cleft lip, and cleft palate. Malformations usually occur early in embryonic development. They often require surgical correction, and are associated with perinatal morbidity. Malformations are widely heterogeneous in their etiology. For example, craniosynostosis (an abnormally shaped skull due to premature fusion of the cranial bones) occurs in at least 90 syndromes (Cohen, 1997).

Deformation refers to an abnormal shape or position of a part of the body caused by mechanical forces in utero. Examples of deformations include limb positioning defects, such as clubfoot or congenital hip dislocation, and minor facial deformities, such as a small chin (micrognathia) or facial asymmetry. Deformations usually occur during the third trimester, and often represent intrauterine molding from mechanical constraint (e.g., breech presentation, decreased or lack of amniotic fluid, multiple births). Most deformations due to these factors spontaneously correct themselves because the infant is no longer subjected to intrauterine constraints. However, deformations secondary to an intrinsic cause (such as abnormal formation of the central nervous system, renal dysfunction, or neuromuscular dysfunction) are associated with neonatal morbidity. These intrinsic factors often have a genetic etiology such as hereditary neuropathies and myopathies or renal malformations.

Disruptions are the result of interference with an originally normal development process. There is extensive clinical variability in disruptions. Examples of a disruption include digit amputation or facial clefting from amniotic bands. Structural abnormalities due to disruptions often have a vascular etiology such as the rare occurrence of limb reduction anomalies following chorionic villus sampling. Maternal factors such as infections and teratogens can be at the root of birth defects from disruptions. The clinician should obtain a detailed pregnancy history regarding the mother of the affected child. For congenital anomalies due to disruptions, the recurrence risk for the parents to have another affected child is usually small.

Although the separation of birth anomalies into the singular categories of malformations, deformations, and disruptions is a valuable clinical tool for determining the etiology of birth defects, the three categories are interrelated. A single extraneous variable can have different physical effects. Decreased amniotic fluid (oligohydramnios) in the third trimester can result in minor deformations (e.g., clubfoot, micrognathia), whereas oligohydramnios in early embryologic development can be related to the disruptive limb-body wall complex (thoracoabdominal wall deficiency with craniofacial anomalies). Micrognathia caused by intrauterine constraint in early fetal development can lead to failure of the tongue to descend resulting in a developmental malformation—cleft palate. The malformation spina bifida may produce leg paralysis leading to the deformations of congential hip dislocation and clubfoot (Cohen, 1997).

Table 4.4 summarizes the general medical-family history questions to pose when there is a family history of one or more birth defects. The medical-family history inquiry is similar for any history of birth anomalies. Brief discussions on three categories of common malformations (cleft lip with and without cleft palate, neural tube defects and congenital heart defects) follow.

Cleft Lip with and without Cleft Palate

Cleft palate (CP) is a different condition from cleft lip with or without cleft palate (CL/P). The formation of the palate and lips do not occur at the same time in embryologic development; consequently, CP and CL/P are associated with different genetic risks (Robinson and Linden, 1993). Associated birth anomalies occur in a significant number of individuals with isolated cleft palate (40%) (Khoury et al., 1997). Between 7 and 13% of individuals with cleft lip are born with associated birth anomalies, as are 11–14% of individuals with both cleft lip and palate (Robinson and Linden, 1993). More than 300 syndromes are associated with cleft lip and palate (Cohen, 1997). Chromosome anomalies, particularly trisomy 13 and trisomy 18, are common causes of CL/P and cleft palate. A medical geneticist should evaluate newborns with a clefting condition to see if a syndrome can be identified. Likewise, individuals with a clefting condition who are interested in genetic risk assess-

TABLE 4.4   Medical-Family History Questions for Congenital Anomalies

Inquiries Related to the Child/Adult With a Birth Variant or Anomaly

- Does the child/adult have:

  Other birth anomalies (particularly of the hands and feet)? Explain.

  Anything unusual about his or her facial appearance, such as unusual placement or appearance of the eyes, nose, mouth, or ears?

  Any birthmarks? If yes, describe their color, number, shape, size, and location.

  Any hearing problems? (If yes, see Section 4.3)

  Any visual problems? (If yes, see Section 4.4)

  Any learning disabilities or problems with schooling? (If yes, see Section 4.5)

  Any delays in achieving developmental milestones?

  Any medical problems, particularly neurological or muscle weakness? Explain.

- Does he or she resemble other family members in appearance?
- Is this person of normal stature? Are the limbs in proportion? (If not, see Section 4.14)

Pregnancy History for the Mother of the Affected Person

- Were there any problems in the pregnancy (e.g., premature rupture of membranes, placental problems)?
- Was the pregnancy full term? Premature?
- What was the fetal presentation at delivery (e.g. breech, vertex)?
- What was the mode of delivery (e.g., a C-section may be an indication of breech presentation or fetal distress)?
- Did the mother have any infections or illnesses during the pregnancy? If so, obtain information about timing during pregnancy.
- Does the mother have any medical problems such as diabetes, cardiovascular disease, or epilepsy?
- Did she take any medications (particularly for seizures) during the pregnancy? If so, obtain specific information about the medication, dosage, and timing.
- Did the mother drink alcohol or use tobacco products? If so, obtain information about usage and timing in pregnancy.
- Did the mother use street drugs (particularly cocaine)? If so, obtain information about usage and timing in pregnancy.
- What were the results of any prenatal testing (such as ultrasound, maternal serum marker testing, amniocentesis, or chorionic villus sampling)?

Family History Questions

- Does anyone have a history of pregnancy losses such as miscarriages or stillbirths?
- Have other babies been born with birth anomalies? If so, describe the defects.
- Does anyone in the family have:

  Mental retardation? (If yes, see Table 4.12)

  A neurological condition? If yes, explain and note the age of onset of symptoms (see Table 4.14)

  Muscle weakness? If yes, explain and note the age of onset of symptoms.

  Hearing loss? If yes, note the severity and age of onset (see Table 4.7)

- Are the parents of the affected individual blood relatives? If so, what is their exact relationship (i.e., the mother's father and the father's father are brothers, therefore the child's parents are first cousins)?

ment for reproductive planning should be offered a genetic evaluation, preferably *prior* to conception.

Cleft lip and palate has been associated with several teratogens in pregnancy including alcohol abuse. The prescription drugs hydantoin, trimethadione, aminopterin, and methotrexate are associated with CL/P. Hyperthermia in the mother (early in pregnancy) and maternal PKU are associated with cleft palate. Amniotic bands can cause a disruption in fetal development resulting in cleft lip. Maternal tobacco use in pregnancy may increase the risk of orofacial clefting through a gene–environment interaction in children with certain alleles of TGF-alpha (transforming growth factor alpha) (Shaw et al., 1996). Some studies suggest that vitamin supplementation with folic acid may help to prevent orofacial clefting (Czeizel et al., 1996; Tolarova and Harris, 1995).

A syndrome commonly associated with cleft lip is Van der Woude syndrome, an autosomal dominant syndrome with reduced penetrance and extremely variable expression such that the clinical manifestations vary from pits in the lower lips to severe cleft lip. Parents of a child with a seemingly isolated cleft lip should be examined for lip pits. If one of the parents has lip pits, than the couple's chance to have another child with a cleft lip is about 26% (not everyone who inherits the gene alteration has clefting). This compares to an approximately 4% recurrence risk if the parents have a normal examination and there is no other family history of clefting (Robinson and Linden, 1993; Tewfik and der Kaloustian, 1997).

Velocardiofacial (DiGeorge) syndrome is an autosomal dominant syndrome characterized by cleft palate, cardiac anomalies (conotruncal), frequent infections, typical facies, and learning disabilities. Velocardiofacial syndrome (VCFS) may be the most common cleft palate syndrome. Shprintzen and colleagues (1985) reported that VCFS accounts for 8.1% of children with palatal clefts.

Most isolated instances of CL/P or cleft palate follow a multifactorial model of causation. Risk of recurrence for the healthy parents of an affected child are gleaned from empirical risk tables, and range from 3–7% for CL/P to 2–5% for cleft palate. A parent with an apparently isolated CL/P has a 2–4% chance to have a child with CL/P, and a parent with cleft palate has a 2–5% chance to have a child with a cleft palate.

Congenital Heart Defects

Congenital heart defects (CHD) are the most common form of birth anomaly, affecting more than 1/200 newborns worldwide (Burn and Goodship, 1997). Between 20% and 45% of infants with a CHD have other noncardiac abnormalities. A specific genetic cause is identified in about one in five children with a cardiac malformation. Usually CHDs occur sporadically, with about 10% occurring as part of a syndrome (Seashore and Wappner, 1996). Congenital heart malformations are associated with close to 200 syndromes. Burn and Goodship (1997) provide a comprehensive list of the syndromes associated with cardiac malformation as well as a listing by major features (e.g., dysmorphic features and mental retardation, limb reduction defects, polydactyly, skeletal defects, ear and eye anomalies, genitourinary defects). Velocardiofacial syndrome (VCFS) is thought to account for 5% of congenital heart anomalies and 20% of outflow defects (VCFS is caused by a 22q deletion that is inherited as an autosomal dominant). A chromosome anomaly (defined as variation from the normal number of chromosomes) should be considered in any newborn (or fetus) with a CHD, especially if the child has other congenital anomalies or dysmorphic features.

There are several known teratogenic influences on the developing heart (Table 4.5). Maternal alcohol use and maternal diabetes are the most significant environmental causes of CHD.

Neural Tube Defects

Neural tube defects (NTD) (e.g., anencephaly, exencephaly, iniencephaly, encephalocele, meningocele and myelomeningocele, spina bifida occulta) are central nervous system birth defects involving problems with closure of the neural tube. Most neural tube defects occur as isolated defects. It is estimated that 50–70% of all neural tube defects would be eliminated if pregnant women were to consume 0.4 mg of folic acid daily. The problem is that the neural tube closes before 28 days after conception, usually before a woman knows she is pregnant. Because as many as

TABLE 4.5   Common Cardiac Teratogens

Teratogenic Agent	Heart Defect[a]
Maternal factors	
Maternal alcohol abuse	VSD, ASD, PDA, double-outlet right ventricle, tetralogy of Fallot
Maternal epilepsy	TGA
Maternal diabetes (particularly if poorly controlled)	TGA, VSD, coarctation of aorta, HLHS
Maternal phenylketonuria (PKU) (poorly controlled)	VSD, PDA, tetralogy of Fallot, HLHS
Maternal rubella	VSD, ASD, PDA, peripheral pulmonary artery stenosis
Maternal systemic lupus erythematosus	Fetal heart block
Drugs	
Androgenic hormones	tetralogy of Fallot, TGA
Hydantoin	VSD
Lithium	ASD, Ebstein anomaly, tricuspid atresia
Retinoic acid/Isotretinoin (Accutane®)/excessive vitamin A	VSD, coarctation of the aorta, HLHS, tetralogy of Fallot, TGA
Thalidomide	ASD, VSD, tetralogy of Fallot, truncus arteriosus
Trimethadione	TGA, HLHS, tetralogy of Fallot
Valproic acid	VSD

[a]ASD = atrial septal defect; HLHS = hypoplastic left heart syndrome; PDA = persistent ductus arteriosus; TGA = transposition of the great arteries; VSD = ventricular septal defect.
Sources: Burn and Goodship, 1996; Sanders, 1996; Robinson and Linden, 1993.

40–50% of pregnancies are unplanned, the Food and Drug Administration mandates supplementation of grains with folic acid. Women who have a previous child with an isolated NTD should consume 4.0 mg of folic acid daily preferably three months before conception and during pregnancy (http://www.cdc.gov/nceh/programs/infants/brthdfct/prevent /ntd_prev.htm, updated 20 Dec. 1996; ACMG, 1998). The total daily intake of folic acid should not exceed 1.0 mg unless prescribed by a physician.

Neural tube defects are often sporadic, but if the child has dysmorphic features with or without other major or minor anomalies, a chromosomal or single gene syndrome should be considered. The secondary medical consequences of a primary neural tube defect (e.g., hydrocephalus, scoliosis, dilated urinary tract, clubfoot) are not considered primary malformations (Tolmie, 1997).

The major teratogenic influences on neural tube defects are valproic acid, poorly controlled insulin-dependent diabetes mellitus, and maternal hyperthermia. These exposures must occur prior to the closure of the neural tube at 28 days in pregnancy.

The Detection of Fetal Anomalies on Routine Ultrasound Examination

Fetal malformations are usually identified serendipitously during a routine ultrasound. Clinicians challenged with making a precise fetal diagnosis are limited by a snapshot glimpse of the fetus, instead of the luxury of the full-system review that can be done after birth. Certainly a family history can assist with attempts at diagnosing a fetal condition; yet the pedigree may not influence *immediate* management decisions. The sonographic finding of any malformation necessitates an immediate discussion about further testing to determine the fetal chromosome pattern.(i.e., by obtaining amniotic fluid or umbilical cord blood). This is true regardless of the parental family history or any potential maternal exposures to fetal teratogens. When a fetal anomaly is detected, it is reasonable to obtain an abbreviated family history from the parents, as is outlined in Table 4.6. A more thorough family history can be initiated once the chromosome results are available. Reviews by Eydoux and Khalife (1997), Sanders et al. (1996), and Snijders and Nicholaides (1996) provide practical approaches to the many differential diagnoses to consider with specific ultrasound findings.

The news of a potential abnormality in what was thought to be a "normal" pregnancy is a crisis for the unsuspecting parents. The parents usually experience shock, worry, grief, guilt, even emotional detachment from the pregnancy, when confronted by this turn of events. They are likely to have little tolerance for the probing questions required for taking an exhaustive three-generation pedigree. The parents, through their fog of grief and worry, may even feel the health professional is asking questions to assign blame (especially with questions about teratogens and consanguinity). Other family members may not know about the pregnancy; inquiring about the extended family may be viewed as a threat to privacy, further compounding the difficulties in obtaining an extensive pedigree.

TABLE 4.6   Minimal Medical-Family History Information to Obtain from the Parents after an Abnormal Fetal Ultrasound

Current Obstetrical History

- What have you been told about the ultrasound findings?
- What is the date of your last menstrual period?
- Have there been any complications during the pregnancy? (e.g., bleeding)
- Have you had other testing during the pregnancy? (e.g., maternal serum screening, prior ultrasounds)
- Is the father of the baby involved with this pregnancy? (Ask this question if he is not present at the visit)
- Was this a planned pregnancy? (If not, the mother may not have had early prenatal care, or the fetus may have been exposed to teratogens before the mother knew she was pregnant)

Past Obstetrical History

- How many pregnancies have you had altogether? (Include miscarriages, terminations of pregnancy, live births, and delivery mode)
- For any pregnancy terminations, was the termination due to a fetal anomaly or a "medical" indication?
- Were any of the pregnancies with a different partner?
- What are your children's ages, and do they have any medical problems?

Mother's Health

- Do you have any health problems? (Specifically inquire about diabetes and high blood pressure, colds, fever, and illnesses in the pregnancy especially if the fetal problems could have a viral etiology)
- Do you take any medications on a regular basis?
- Have you taken any prescription or over-the-counter drugs or herbal medicines during the pregnancy?
- Are you taking prenatal vitamins?
- Do you use any recreational drugs? (Note amount and timing)
- Do you smoke or chew tobacco?
- How much alcohol have you had during the pregnancy? (Note quantity, type of beverage, and how often)

Father's Health

- Does the father of the baby have any medical problems?
- Has the father of the baby had children or pregnancies (including miscarriages) with any previous partners? Do his children have any medical problems?

Maternal and Paternal Family History

- Is there anyone in your family, or the family of the baby's father, who have had a baby with a birth defect, mental retardation, or learning problems?
- Does anyone in the family have any major medical problems?
- Are the two of you related as blood relatives? For example, are you cousins?
- Has anyone in either family had a miscarriage, a stillborn baby, or a baby that died?

Is there anything I have not asked you about, or anything else in your family history that you think is important for me to know about?

*If the patient answers yes to any of these questions, a more extensive family history is warranted, asking directed questions as appropriate.

4.3 DEAFNESS/HEARING LOSS

Given that nearly 50% of individuals have significant hearing impairment by age 80, uncovering a family history of hearing loss is not surprising. The prevalence of severe hearing loss in children under the age of three years is approximately 2/1,000 births (Khoury et al., 1997). About 4/1,000 children under age 19 years are hearing impaired (Fischel-Ghodsian and Falk, 1997). Genetic factors account for about half of all hearing loss. Over 60 different genes causing nonsyndromal and syndromal deafness have been discovered (Van Camp and Smith, 1998). Acquired causes and unknown reasons equally subdivide the remaining etiological factors in hearing loss (Khoury et al., 1997).

Because 90% of deaf individuals have children with other deaf individuals, careful genetic counseling for these couples is important (Cohen and Gorlin, 1995). With more than 400 inherited syndromes associated with hearing loss, determining the etiology of hearing loss for an individual or family often proves quite a conundrum, particularly because about 90% of individuals with congenital hearing loss have hearing parents (Cohen and Gorlin, 1995). Nonsyndromic deafness has no other signs or symptoms and accounts for the majority (~70%) of hearing loss (Tewfik et al., 1997). Among those with hereditary hearing loss, estimates are that 60–80% is autosomal recessive, 23–36% is autosomal dominant, and about 2–4% is X-linked (Cohen and Gorlin, 1995). Although mitochondrial inheritance is a small contributor to the overall prevalence of hearing loss, sensorineural hearing loss is an extremely common finding in several mitochondrial myopathies (see Table 2.6).

Of nonsyndromic hearing loss, autosomal recessive mutations account for the majority (75–85%), particularly in profound prelingual (before speech) hearing loss. Mutations in a gene called connexin 26 or nonsyndromic neurosensory deafness (DFNB1) probably account for 20% of all childhood hereditary hearing loss (Kelley et al., 1998). Autosomal dominant inheritance is more often seen with postlingual hearing loss, and with moderate or progressive hearing loss. An autosomal dominant pattern of inheritance is the etiology of 15–25% of nonsyndromic hearing loss. Only 1–2% of nonsyndromic inheritance is attributed to X-linked inheritance, and less than 1% to mitochondrial mutations (Van Camp and Smith, 1998).

With more than 60 different genes causing nonsyndromal and syndromal hearing loss, it is easy to confuse the syndrome nomenclature. Nonsyndromic deafness is abbreviated DFN followed by the inheritance pattern (A for autosomal dominant, B for autosomal recessive, and no notation for X-linked) and a number indicating the order the gene was discovered (e.g., DFNA11, DFNB1, DFN4). Syndromic hearing loss is named after the researchers who described the syndrome (e.g., Waardenburg syndrome), or by descriptive terms (e.g., branchio-oto-renal syndrome).

Individuals with chromosome anomalies often have hearing impairment (Tewfik et al., 1997). Although being conscious of this association is important for maximizing learning opportunities for these individuals, hearing loss is rarely a presenting clinical feature in recognizing children with chromosome anomalies, nor is hearing loss prominent in their family histories.

The questions to ask in obtaining a medical-family history for deafness are extensive (see Table 4.7) because almost any organ system can be involved in syndromic deafness. There are six major parameters that help to classify hearing loss (Cohen and Gorlin, 1995; Fischel-Ghodsian and Falk, 1996):

1. Severity of the hearing loss.
2. Type of deafness.
3. Deafness associated with other features (syndromic deafness) versus isolated (undifferentiated) nonsyndromic deafness.
4. Age of onset (congenital/prelingual, and postlingual childhood or adult onset).
5. Progressive versus nonprogressive hearing impairment.
6. Acquired (either prenatal or postnatal) versus genetic.

Medical record documentation of hearing studies and medical problems is essential for accurate genetic assessment. Numerous syndromes involve hearing loss and eye disorders, so it is important to obtain records of ophthalmologic evaluations. Renal anomalies are also frequently associated with hearing loss. The branchio-oto-renal syndrome (BOR) is seen in 2% of deaf children. Excellent reviews of the syndromes and conditions associated with hereditary deafness can be found in Cremers (1998), Gorlin et al. (1995), Tewfik et al. (1997), and Van Camp and Smith's The Hereditary Hearing Loss Homepage (URL: http://dnalab-www.uia.ac.be/dnalab/hhh, updated 5-Nov-1998).

Providing genetic assessment to a deaf individual or couple can be challenging at many levels (Israel et al., 1996). A hearing health provider may have trouble obtaining a medical-family history from a deaf client, because of communication barriers. Deaf individuals may use any combination of skills to communicate, such as a "signed language" like American or British Sign Language (ASL and BSL, respectively), lip reading, a tactile communicator (for a deaf–blind individual), writing on paper, or using a laptop computer. Phone conversation between an individual with hearing loss and the hearing health provider can be accessed through a TTY message-relay system. The service operator relays, word for word, the communication between the message typed by the deaf person to the hearing person, and vice versa. A certified ASL interpreter (preferably one with medical knowledge) should interpret during clinical visits.

A hearing-impaired individual may have difficulty communicating with his or her hearing relatives. Thus, he or she may have limited knowledge about the health of many family members. The clinician may be able to obtain additional family history information by contacting a hearing family member directly. In this instance, it is important to respect the confidentiality of the nonhearing client.

From the perspective of the hearing health professional, the translated "speech"or rapidly scrawled words of the nonhearing patient may seem terse and choppy. American Sign Language is not merely a codification of English; ASL does not directly translate into English. Difficulties with translation are compounded by

TABLE 4.7 Medical-Family History Questions for Deafness/Hearing Loss

- What is the type of hearing loss?
    Conductive (external ear defects involving pinna and/or outer ear canal, and/or middle
      ear defects involving tympanic membrane, ossicles or eustachian tube)
    Sensorineural (perceptive or neuronal type involving inner ear/cochlear defects)
    Mixed
- How severe is the hearing loss?
    Mild (20–40 dB)
    Moderate (40–60 dB)
    Severe (60–80 dB)
    Profound (>80 dB)
- What is the hearing impaired individual's method of communication?
    Sign language
    Lip reading
    Tactile (for deaf–blind)
    Speech (note that nasal speech suggests velopharyngeal insufficiency)
- At what age was the hearing loss detected?
    Prelingual (onset prior to speech development)
    Postlingual (onset after speech development)
- Is the hearing loss progressive or nonprogressive?
- Has the individual had chronic exposure to noise? (occupational or environmental)
- Has the individual had any chronic diseases, or trauma to the ear?
    Chronic ear infections
    Meningitis
    Mastoiditis
    Kernicterus (bilirubin encephalopathy)
    Myxedema (hypothyroidism)
- Did the individual's mother have any illnesses or problems during her pregnancy? (include
  timing of exposure)
    Rubella
    Alcohol (amount)
    Cytomegalovirus
    Toxoplasmosis
    Retinoic acid
    Quinine
    Maternal diabetes
    Oligohydramnios (possible fetal kidney problem)
- Has the individual had any problems with learning? (inquire about special education) (see
  Section 4.5)
    Mental retardation
      Progressive
      Nonprogressive
    Learning disabilities
- Does the person have any unusual physical features?
    Eyes (physical)
      Placement
        Hypertelorism (wide spaced)
        Hypotelorism (close together)
      Shape (small, absent, down-slanting)
      Eyelid
        Coloboma (notched) (common in mandibulofacial dysostosis)
        Ptosis (droopy)

(continued)

TABLE 4.7   *(continued)*

Coloring
    Heterochromia (different colored) (seen in Waardenburg syndrome)
    Blue sclerae (white of eyes) (common in the osteogenesis imperfectas and
        Ehlers–Danlos syndrome VI/Kyphoscoliosis type)
Visual problems (include age at onset) and note any treatments (see Section 4.4)
    Progressive
    Nonprogressive
    Glaucoma
    Cataracts (see Tables 4.9 and 4.10)
    Retinitis pigmentosa (frequently associated with syndromic hearing loss, particularly
        with the Usher syndromes)
Ears (external anomalies are extremely common in syndromic hearing loss)
    Physical shape and size (describe: e.g., cupped, crumpled)
    Absent
    Placement (e.g., low-set, rotated)
    Ear tags (common in oculo-auriculo-vertebral dysplasia)
    Ear pits (common in branchio-oto-renal syndrome)
Nose
    Unusual shape
        Pear or bulbous (common in the tricho-rhino-phalangeal syndrome)
        Depressed nasal bridge
        Wide nasal bridge
    Inability to smell (Kallman syndrome)
Mouth
    Cleft lip
    Cleft palate
    High arched palate
    Lip pits (seen in Van der Woude syndrome)
Chin
    Micrognathia (small) (seen in Treacher–Collins syndrome)
    Prognathic (large)
Face
    Asymmetric
    Unusual shape (e.g, long, seen in tricho-rhino-phalangeal syndrome; triangular, in the
        osteogenesis imperfectas)
    Coarsening of facial features (common in lysosomal storage disorders)
Head
    Microcephaly (small)
    Macrocephaly (large)
Hair
    White streaks (don't mistake artificial coloring!) (seen in Waardenburg syndrome)
    Sparse or patchy
    Coarse (common in storage disorders)
Teeth
    Conical
    Malocclusion
    Discoloration
    "Brittle" (common in osteogenesis imperfecta)

(continued)

TABLE 4.7   *(continued)*

Hands and feet
    Short fingers/toes (brachydactyly)
    Long fingers/toes (arachnodactyly)
    Syndactyly (webbed or fused)
    Absent, rotated, misshapen thumb(s)
    Polydactyly (extra fingers/toes)
    Other digit anomalies
- Does the person have other health problems?
    Cardiovascular
        Conduction defects (common in Jervell and Lange–Nielsen syndrome)
        Congenital heart defects (describe anomaly)
    Gastrointestinal
        Enlarged liver or spleen (common in lysosomal storage diseases)
    Renal anomalies (common in Alport syndrome and branchio-oto-renal syndrome)
    Skeletal
        Tall stature
        Short stature (common in many skeletal dysplasias)
        Limbs proportionate
        Limbs disproportionate
        Scoliosis
        Congenital hip dislocation
        Multiple fractures (common in osteogenesis imperfecta)
        Loose joints
    Skin
        Unusual birthmarks (describe)
        Albinism
        Scaling/icthyosis
        Branchial cysts/fistulas (present on lower neck) (seen in branchio-oto-renal
            syndrome)
    Neurological (note age at onset)
        Gait problems (common in Charcot–Marie–Tooth, Friedreich ataxia, mitochondrial
            diseases, and several rare ataxia syndromes)
        Brain "tumors" (describe) (common in neurofibromatosis type 2)
        Muscle weakness
        Spasticity
        Seizures (see Section 4.8)
        Stroke-like episodes
        Episodic vomiting/headaches (common in metabolic and mitochondrial disorders)
        Dementia (Note age at onset, see Section 4.9)
        Movement disorder
    Endocrine
        Diabetes (see Section 4.15)
        Thyroid disease (seen in Pendred syndrome)
    Fertility problems
        Hypogonadism (seen in Kallman syndrome, Norrie disease)
- Are the parents of the child blood relatives? (e.g., first cousins or more closely related)

Sources: Gorlin et al., 1990, 1995; Tewfik et al., 1997.

the fact that many deaf individuals have had barriers to quality education. For reasons such as these, unfortunately, a hearing health professional may falsely perceive that the deaf individual is "slow."

Often individuals with hearing impairment consider themselves "Deaf"—a descriptive name for a unifying culture, not a medical label describing a handicapping condition (Israel et al., 1996; Middleton et al., 1998). Health professionals need to determine the client's preferred terminology for describing his or her hearing difficulties (e.g., hearing impairment, deafness, hard-of-hearing), and use this terminology in discussion with the client. Couples in which one or both individuals are deaf may have few concerns about having a child who is also deaf. In fact, they may worry about raising a child who is hearing (Middleton et al., 1998). The nonhearing couple may take offense to clinical lingo describing "risks" of having a "hearing-*impaired*," "abnormal," or "affected" child as compared to a "normal" hearing child. The clinician should choose words reflecting "chances" over risks, and describe children as "hearing" or "nonhearing" (Cohen and Gorlin, 1995; Fischel-Ghodsain and Falk, 1997; Israel et al., 1996).

4.4 VISION IMPAIRMENT

With better control of nutrition and of maternal and childhood infections (such as smallpox and maternal rubella), inherited disorders account for a large fraction of congenital and childhood visual impairment. Estimates are that half of all visual impairment before the age of 45 years has a genetic etiology; all inheritance patterns are represented including single gene, mitochondrial, and chromosomal (Robinson and Linden, 1993). Obtaining medical documentation of the type and degree of visual disturbance is absolutely essential to provide genetic counseling. Retinal dystrophies are the most common form of genetic blindness (accounting for more than 50%) (Aldred et al., 1994). More than 200 inherited disorders involve retinal degeneration (usually presenting as night blindness and eventual loss of central vision) (Heckenlively and Daiger, 1997). Conversely, 10% of all inherited disorders involve the retina directly or indirectly (Heckenlively and Daiger, 1997). The important medical-family history features to document when an individual has congenital blindness or later-onset visual loss are reviewed in Table 4.8.

Early-onset Cataracts

Approximately 1/250 infants are born with a cataract (Robinson and Linden, 1993). Worldwide, 10% of all blindness is attributed to congenital cataracts (Rabinowitz et al., 1997). Cataracts seem to be involved in the aging process, for all humans will develop cataracts that can impair vision if they live to an advanced age. The upper age limit that is considered "early" for the onset of cataracts is debatable (R. Kalina, personal communication).

Determining the significance of a family history of cataracts can be sorted by the age of presentation of the cataracts (congenital; infancy, <12 months; childhood, 1–15 years; and adult, >15 years). Approximately 70–75% of congenital cataracts

TABLE 4.8   The Medical-Family History Approach to Visual Loss

- What was the person's age at the onset of blindness or visual loss?
- Document with ophthalmologic records the area of visual pathology (some conditions will overlap in more than one area):
    Retina (e.g., retinitis pigmentosa, macular degeneration, retinoblastoma)
    Choroid (e.g., choroideremia)
    Optic nerve or disc (e.g., atrophy, hypoplasia)
    Lens (e.g., cataract, ectopia lentis)
    Eyeball or globe (e.g., high myopia, glaucoma, structural defect such as microphthalmos or anophthalmos)
    Iris (uvea) and uveal tract (e.g., aniridia or iris hypoplasia, coloboma, chorioretinitis)
    Nystagmus (common in disorders of hypopigmentation such as albinism)
- Is the visual disturbance bilateral or unilateral? (bilateral disease is more likely to have a genetic etiology)
- Did the mother of the person with visual impairment have any infections during the pregnancy?
- Are the parents of the person with visual impairment related as cousins (or more closely)? (suggestive of autosomal recessive inheritance)
- Does the person (or other family members) have other diseases or medical conditions? Focus on:
    Dysmorphic features with or without other birth anomalies (see Section 4.2)
    Hearing loss (see Section 4.3). The various forms of the autosomal recessive Usher syndrome (retinitis pigmentosa with sensorineural hearing loss) account for 8% of profound deafness in children. Among the deaf–blind population, RP has a prevalence estimated at 50% (Gorlin et al., 1995)
    Mental retardation or learning disabilities (see Section 4.5)
    Neurological disease (see Section 4.7)
    Dementia (see Section 4.9)
    Pigmentary and skin abnormalities
    Short stature (see Section 4.14)
    Diabetes (see Section 4.15)
    Reproductive anomalies including hypogonadism (see Section 4.16)

Source: Arnould and Hussels, 1997; Gorlin et al., 1995.

are nongenetic in etiology. Worldwide, maternal infections (e.g., rubella, varicella, toxoplasmosis) are an important cause of congenital cataracts. Diabetes mellitus is a frequent fundamental metabolic factor in the development of childhood cataracts. Presenile cataracts can be secondary to an underlying lens anomaly, which may or may not have a hereditary etiology (Rabinowitz et al., 1997) such as:

1. *Ectopia lentis* (dislocated lens). Ectopia lentis can occur as a result of a traumatic blow to the head, as an isolated hereditary condition (autosomal dominant or recessive), or as a feature of an inherited syndrome (such as Marfan syndrome or homocystinuria).

2. *Iris coloboma* (notching). Iris colobomas are associated with several chromosomal anomalies and CHARGE association. Colobomas may occur after an injury or surgery.

3. *Multiple lenticonus* (a bulge in the front or back of the lens).

4. *Retinal degeneration associated with retinitis pigmentosa* (usually develops after the age of 30 years).

Several chromosomal syndromes are associated with the development of cataracts at a young age (Rabinowitz et al., 1997). Early age at onset of cataracts is seen in several inborn errors of metabolism (see Table 4.9) in which the underlying defect is in cholesterol synthesis or metabolism (e.g., galactosemia, manosidosis, neuraminidase deficiency, Lowe syndrome, Wilson disease, untreated PKU, Smith–Lemli–Opitz syndrome, Zellweger syndrome, cerebrotendinous xanthomatosis, mevalonic aciduria) (Berry and Bennett, 1998; Rabinowitz et al., 1997).

TABLE 4.9   Examples of Hereditary and Environmental Syndromes Associated with Early-Onset Cataracts

Age at Presentation	Syndrome	Inheritance Pattern[a]	Other Cardinal Features[a]
Birth	Lowe (oculocerebrorenal) syndrome	XL	Short stature, sebaceous cysts, MR, hypotonia, dysmorphic features, renal disease
	Zellweger syndrome	AR	Seizures, dysmorphic features, joint contractures, hepatomegaly, hypotonia
	Rhizomelic chondrodysplasia punctata	AR	MR, proximal limb shortening, ichthyosis
	Cockayne syndrome B	AR	LD/MR (progressive), dysmorphic features, hearing loss, retinal degeneration, premature aging, short stature
	Warburg syndrome	AR	MR, severe brain malformations, other eye anomalies, congenital muscular dystrophy
	Marshall syndrome	AD	Hearing loss, dysmorphic features, skeletal anomalies, ectodermal dysplasia
	Oculomandibulofacial syndrome (Hallerman–Streiff)	?	Dysmorphic features including characteristic beaked nose, variable LD/MR, dental anomalies, dermatologic findings
Newborn (1 wk–1 mo)	Galactosemia	AR	Successful dietary intervention with lactose-free diet but may still have LD, growth delays, ovarian failure; identified by newborn screening in the United States
	Fetal rubella	Maternal infection	MR, deafness, chorioretinitis, glaucoma, patent ductus arteriosis, peripheral pulmonic stenosis, myocardial disease

(continued)

TABLE 4.9   *(continued)*

Age at Presentation	Syndrome	Inheritance Pattern[a]	Other Cardinal Features[a]
	Fetal varicella	Maternal infection	MR, seizures, chorioretinitis, limb/digit anomalies, growth deficiency
Infancy (1–12 mo)	Galactokinase deficiency	AR	Cataracts may be only manifestation
	Lysosomal storage diseases	AR, XL	Coarsening facies, MR/LD, hepatosplenomegaly, bony changes (dysostosis multiplex)
	Smith–Lemli–Opitz syndrome	AR	MR, short stature, dysmorphic features, genitourinary and limb anomalies
Childhood (1–5 y)	Wilson disease	AR	Liver disease from copper accumulation, psychiatric disease, neurological deterioration
	Neurofibromatosis II	AD	Hearing loss, vestibular schwannomas, brain tumors (meningomas, gliomas)
	Stickler syndrome	AD	LD, dysmorphic features, retinal detachment, myopia, hypotonia, hyperextensible joints, skeletal anomalies, cleft palate
	Incontinentia pigmenti	XL (lethal in males)	MR/LD, neurological deficits, skin lesions which are replaced by hyper-pigmented/hypopigmented areas, dental anomalies
	Pseudohypoparathyroidism	XL	LD, short stature, brachydactyly, hypocalcemia
Adulthood (>15 y)	Myotonic muscular dystrophy	AD	Myotonia, muscle weakness, ptosis
	Cerebrotendinous xanthomatosis	AR	Xanthomas, thickening tendons, spasticity, dysarthria, dementia and neurological deterioration, cardiovascular disease
	Alport syndrome	AD, XL	Sensorineural hearing loss, renal disease
	Werner syndrome	AR	Characteristic dermatologic pathology and facies, short stature, hypogonadism, premature aging

[a]Abbreviations: LD = learning disabled; MR = mental retardation; AD = autosomal dominant; AR = autosomal recessive; XL = X-linked; ? = unknown etiology.
Sources: Clarke, 1996; Jones, 1997; Rabinowitz et al., 1997; Saudubray and Charpentier, 1995; Sybert, 1997.

TABLE 4.10 Medical-Family History Queries for Cataracts

- At what age were the cataracts diagnosed?
- Are the cataracts in both eyes?
- Does the person have other problems with his or her eyes? (obtain ophthalmologic records)
- Does the person with the cataracts have a history of diabetes?
- Does the person have any unusual facial or physical features?
- What is the height of the person?
- Is the person unusually tall or short compared to other family members? (record parental and sibling heights)
- Did the mother of the person with cataracts have any infections in pregnancy?
- Does the person with cataracts, or his or her family members, have:
  Other medical problems? Explain
  Any unusual skin findings? Describe
  Mental retardation or learning disabilities? (see Section 4.5)
  Hearing loss? (note severity and age at onset, see Section 4.3)
  Heart disease? (see section 4.11)
  Any muscle weakness?
  Any neurological problems (such as slurred speech, unsteady gait, seizures)? (see Section 4.7)
- Psychiatric disease, dementia, or significant behavioral problems? (see Section 4.10)
  Any kidney disease? (see Section 4.13)
- Do other people in the family have cataracts or other eye diseases?

Because multiple rare syndromes feature early-onset cataracts (see Table 4.9), referral to a medical geneticist is recommended. Table 4.10 reviews the family-medical history questions for cataracts.

4.5 MENTAL RETARDATION

Mental retardation is not something you have, like blue eyes or a bad heart, nor is it something you are, like short or thin. It is not a medical disorder or a mental disorder . . . Mental retardation reflects the "fit" between the capabilities of individuals and the structure and expectations of their environment.
—American Association on Mental Retardation (1992)

Concern about a family member with mental retardation is frequently the impetus for a person or couple to seek genetic counseling. Approximately 0.5–1% of newborns have conditions associated with moderate to severe retardation (an IQ less than 50) (Bundey, 1997). Varying degrees of mental retardation affect between 2.0 and 3.0% of the general population (Bundey, 1997; Robinson and Linden, 1993). Severe mental retardation is more likely to have a genetic etiology (30–40% are the result of single gene or chromosomal disorders) than milder forms of mental retardation (Bundey, 1997; Robinson and Linden, 1993). Chromosomal syndromes are responsible for the majority of the identifiable causes of severe mental retardation (See Table 2.1 for family history features suggestive of a chromosomal syndrome). Down syndrome is believed to be the etiology for one in three of all individuals with moderate mental retardation. Twenty-five to 50% of all mental retardation is attributed to X-linked genes, with fragile X syndrome contributing to approximately 30–50% of all individuals with X-linked mental retardation (Sutherland and Mulley, 1997). Molecular testing for fragile X should be considered in any male or female with unexplained mental retardation (in the absence of minor or major malformations) (Jones, 1997). Sutherland and Mulley (1997) provide an excellent and comprehensive review of more than 100 X-linked syndromes associated with mental retardation. Autosomal recessive or X-linked inborn errors of metabolism are responsible for about 5% of all severe postnatal mental retardation (Jones, 1997). See Table 4.11 for clinical and family history features suggestive of an inherited inborn error of metabolism.

TABLE 4.11   Features Suggestive of a Metabolic Genetic Disorder

- Failure to thrive
- Hypotonia
- Loss of developmental milestones
- Mental retardation/global developmental delay
- Head circumference which is normal at birth then fails to follow the growth curve
- Progressive worsening of symptoms
- Periodic symptoms
- Episodic vomiting
- Metabolic acidosis
- Episodic hypoglycemia
- Intermittent coma
- Chronic diarrhea
- Recurrent infections
- Symptoms brought on by infectious illness or fasting
- Symptoms began with weaning
- Abnormal behavior (irritable, impulsive, aggressive, hyperactive, self-mutilation)
- Seizures
- Cataracts in infancy or childhood
- Hair anomalies:
    Excessive body hair (hirsute)
    Brittle, fragile hair
    Stiff, kinky, or coarse hair
    Sparse or absent hair (alopecia)
- Coarsening of facial features
- Dysostosis multiplex
- Enlarged liver and/or spleen
- Unusual odor (particularly when ill):
    sweaty feet, cheese (isovaleric acidemia, glutaric acidemia type 2
    rancid, fishy, rotten cabbage (tyrosinemia)
    musty, mousy (untreated PKU)
    sweet (maple syrup urine disease)
    fishy (trimethylaminuria)
    hops, beer, dried celery (methionine malabsorption)
- Poor feeding
- Unusual dietary pattern (e.g., avoids protein)
- Parental consanguinity
- Autosomal recessive or X-linked inheritance patterns are typical

Sources: Berry and Bennett, 1998; Bundey, 1997; Clarke,1996; Lashley FR, 1998; Saudubray and Charpentier, 1995.

Be wary of the language you use when inquiring about a family member with developmental disabilities. Many families and disability advocates feel "mental retardation" is a derogatory term. Instead, they may prefer descriptions such as "learning disabled," "mentally or educationally challenged," "slow learner," "special needs," even "differently abled" (Finucane, 1998). It is appropriate to say the "child with mental retardation" but not the "mentally retarded child." The use of suitable descriptors of intellectual functioning is extremely important when discussing reproductive risks and choices with a man, woman, or couple with mental delays. Journalist Michael Bérubé, the parent of a child with Down syndrome, represents the thoughts of many disability activists regarding sensitivity toward the "language of mental retardation" when he writes:

> I'm told that intelligence has obvious survival value, since organisms with a talent for information processing 'naturally' beat out their competitors for food, water, and condos, but human history doesn't convince me that *our* brand of intelligence is just what the world was waiting for.
>
> —Michael Bérubé (1996)

Mild mental retardation may "run in the family," and have both an environmental and genetic etiology. Asking about the parents' mental abilities is important. Although it is often difficult to determine the cause of mild mental retardation, a family history of "normal intelligence" can be very reassuring to the inquiring family member.

It is not unusual for a person with mild mental retardation to consider childbearing. A myriad of environmental, social, and family history variables complicate the assessment of reproductive risks for these individuals (Finucane, 1998). Individuals with mild mental retardation often live under impoverished conditions, adding potential environmental deprivation to the at-risk child's developmental milieu. There is a good likelihood that the partner of the affected individual is also learning disabled. This leads to the added complication of needing to make a genetic risk assessment based on two parents affected with learning disabilities which most likely have different etiologies (Finucane, 1998). The incidence of sexual abuse perpetrated against women with developmental disabilities is high. Because a significant proportion of this abuse is committed by blood relatives, there can be the added component of risk for autosomal recessive conditions because of parental incest (Finucane, 1998).

There are many unique issues in providing genetic counseling to individuals with mild mental retardation. The potential parent with learning disabilities may be less concerned about having a child "like me," who also has learning delays, than having a child with physical birth defects (Finucane, 1998). These individuals may be unreliable family historians as well as concrete thinkers who may have difficulty conceptualizing the multitude of facts and figures that are traditionally reviewed in a typical genetic counseling visit. Finucane suggests that the content of such counseling should shift from "facts to feelings" (1998).

When a family history of mental retardation is identified, there are several key historical questions than can help with identification of syndromes and assist with determining recurrence risks. These family history features are summarized in Table 4.12. A simple question to begin with is, *"What diagnostic testing has been done?"* Any child or person with unexplained mental retardation and dysmorphic features should have a chromosome study, particularly if there is a family history of mental retardation and miscarriages (suggesting a chromosome translocation). Individuals born before the 1970s may not have had a banded chromosome study. If an adult with features characteristic of a chromosomal syndrome had a normal chromosome study prior to the early 1990s, it is worth redoing the cytogenetic study using more sophisticated techniques. A normal chromosome study does not eliminate a genetic diagnosis. *"Were any metabolic studies done?"* (such as plasma amino acids, urine organic acids, lactate, or pyruvate). *"Has any neurological testing been done?"* (including brain imaging). Major brain malformations are more likely to have a genetic etiology than are minor structural abnormalities (Bundey, 1997).

"How severe is the learning disability? Do you have the results of any formal developmental testing?" About 30–40% of individuals with severe mental retardation have a single gene or chromosomal disorder, whereas mild mental retardation accounts for about 10% of such cases (Bundey, 1997). Severely aberrant mental development is usually clearly identified by 3 to 6 months of age. Documentation of actual IQ scores from affected family members is important. In the absence of medical records, descriptive information about the individual is useful. For example, *"What life skills does the person have?"* (e.g., feeding and dressing self, the ability to make change, living on own, driving a car or taking a bus, reading).

"Were the problems present from birth?" Developmental delays noted from birth or shortly thereafter suggest a teratogenic exposure in pregnancy, or a chromosomal problem. *"Are the delays remaining static or progressing? If progressive, at what age did the changes begin?"* Normal development, followed by a loss of developmental milestones or progressive decline in school performance, is suggestive of an inherited biochemical disorder (usually autosomal recessive or X-linked recessive; refer to Table 4.11) or a mitochondrial disorder. Persons with chromosomal aneuploidy usually do not regress in their development. Of course, other causes of developmental delay and failure to thrive that should not be overlooked include severe malnutrition, abuse, and neglect. Apparent regression may be attributed to environmental factors such as poorly controlled seizure activity, overmedication with anticonvulsants, intercurrent illness, emotional problems, or depression (Clarke, 1996).

"Were there problems in pregnancy or with birth? Was the child full term? Did the mother take any medications during pregnancy? Does the mother have any medical problems?" Answers to these questions can help determine whether the child's delays are due to genetic or environmental causes (Robinson and Linden, 1993) such as the following:

- Maternal factors (e.g., maternal PKU, maternal myotonic muscular dystrophy)
- Teratogens (e.g., alcohol and/or recreational drugs, fetal hydantoin syndrome)
- Prematurity

TABLE 4.12   Features to Document In the Medical-Family History When a Family Member Has Mental Retardation.

- Severity of mental retardation (DSM IV-Classification)
    Mild (IQ 50–55 to approximately 70)
    Moderate (IQ 35–40 to 50–55)
    Severe (IQ 20–25 to 35–40)
    Profound (IQ < 20–25)
- The age the delays were noted
- Static or progressive mental impairment
- Intellectual abilities of parents of affected child
- Pregnancy and health history of affected child's mother:
    Full gestation or premature
    Traumatic delivery or asphyxiation (e.g., cord accident)
    Teratogenic exposure
        Specifically ask about alcohol and recreational drugs
        Seizure medications
    Maternal infections (syphilis, rubella, toxoplasmosis, cytomegalovirus, HIV, herpes simplex)
    Maternal disease (e.g., PKU, myotonic dystrophy)
- History suggestive of early postnatal trauma (abuse, neglect, severe malnutrition)
- Any episodes of severe childhood illness including:
    Recurrent infections
    Episodic vomiting
    Intermittent coma
    Episodes of hypoglycemia
    Chronic diarrhea
- Anything unusual about the person's dietary pattern
- Unusual body odor, particularly when ill
- Abnormal behavior
- Hearing deficits (type and severity)
- Speech deficits (type and severity)
- Vision deficits (type and severity)
- Height of the individual, and height of parents and siblings
- Birth anomalies
- Physical and dysmorphic features
    Head size (microcephalic or macrocepahlic)
    Eyes
        Unusual placement
        Abnormal movements
    Ears
        Large or unusually shaped
    Face
        Dysmorphic features
        Coarsening of facial features
    Hair
        Patchy, sparse, balding
        Unusual texture (brittle, kinky)
        Excessive body hair
- Unusual skin pigmentation
- Skeletal anomalies
- Joint laxity
- Enlarged liver or spleen
- Large testes

(continued)

TABLE 4.12 (continued)

- Neurological/neuromuscular findings
  Seizures
  Weakness
  Hypotonia or hypertonia
  Gait disturbances
  Involuntary movements
- Family history of:
  Mental retardation/learning disabilities
  Miscarriages
  Multiple birth defects
- Parental consanguinity

Sources: Bundey, 1997; Sutherland and Mulley, 1997.

- Prenatal or perinatal infections or illness
- Birth trauma (e.g., intracerebral hemorrhage)
- Asphyxia (e.g., abruptio placentae, cord prolapse, meconium aspiration)

Children with mental retardation secondary to a prenatal infection (such as rubella, cytomegalic virus, and toxoplasmosis) usually have one or more of the following features: microcephaly, chorioretinitis, prenatal onset growth deficiency, hepatosplenomegaly, neonatal petechiae, jaundice, and deafness (Jones, 1997). Family lore often focuses on birth trauma or drug use in pregnancy as the cause of mental retardation in a family member; obtaining prenatal and birth records can help illuminate whether or not this is a factor in the etiology of an individual's mental delays.

"Did the parents of the individual with learning disabilities have any problems in school? Were they ever in special classes to provide extra help in learning? What types of employment has either parent had? Have other people in the family required extra assistance with learning?" The answers to these questions will give you an idea of the intellectual abilities of the parents of the affected individual or if there is a family history of learning disabilities.

"Has the person had episodes of severe illness requiring hospitalization? Has the individual had episodes of excessive vomiting, coma, or low blood sugar (hypoglycemia)? Has the individual been hospitalized for frequent infections or chronic diarrhea?" Any of these symptoms can be seen in inborn errors of metabolism (Table 4.11).

"Does the person have poor feeding or an unusual dietary pattern?" Avoidance of certain foods (particularly protein) can be a symptom of some of the inborn errors of metabolism (Table 4.11). Excessive eating can be seen in Prader–Willi syndrome (imprinting/microdeletion). *"Does the person have an unusual body odor, particularly when he or she is ill?"* A few of the inborn errors of metabolism are associated with a specific body odor (Table 4.11).

"Are there extreme or unusual behavioral problems?" Destructive behavior may indicate a biochemical genetics problem such as Sanfilippo syndrome or

Lesch–Nyhan syndrome (both autosomal recessive), or Hunter syndrome (X-linked recessive). Mental illness is seen in some of the other autosomal recessive enzyme deficiency disorders including homocystinuria, methylene tetrahydrofolate reductase deficiency, and Krabbe disease. Outbursts of inappropriate laughter may be seen in Angelman syndrome (imprinting/microdeletion). Boys with X-linked adrenoleukodystrophy may present with gait disturbances associated with irritability, withdrawal, obsessive behaviors, and school failure (Clarke, 1996). Schizophrenic-like symptoms can be seen in individuals with velocardiofacial syndrome and other chromosomal syndromes.

"Does the person look the same or different from other family members? Would you be able to tell from a photograph that there is something different about him/her?" Many syndromes with mental retardation have associated dysmorphic features. By inquiring if the person in question has facial features similar to others in the family, it may help you discern whether or not the characteristics are just a familial variation or a unique syndromic feature. Pictures from a family gathering are invaluable.

"How tall is this individual? What are the heights of his or her parents and brothers and sisters?" Unusual stature (particularly short stature) is a feature of many syndromes associated with mental retardation/learning disabilities.

"Does the person with mental retardation/learning disabilities have any birth anomalies or are there birth malformations in other family members? Does the person or other family members have other medical problems (including hearing, speech, or visual deficits)?"

"Is there anything unusual about the person's hair; for example, is it unusually coarse, curly, or brittle? Is the hair absent, patchy, or sparse?" Many syndromes are associated with mental retardation and hair anomalies (Sybert, 1997). Several of the inborn errors of metabolism are associated with differences in the texture and/or fullness of scalp hair.

"Are there any unusual birthmarks or skin problems?" Cutaneous manifestations and varying degrees of mental retardation are associated with at least 50 recognized syndromes (and an endless array of published case reports) (Sybert, 1997 and personal communication; Jones, 1997). Neurofibromatosis 1 is associated with café au lait spots, learning disabilities, and sometimes a large head. Tuberous sclerosis complex is associated with hypopigmented macules ("ashleaf" spots), and angiofibromas clustering on the face, cheeks, nose, and mouth, and shagreen patches (pink, yellow, or whitish plaques). Telangiectasias are a major feature of ataxia telangiectasia.

"Are there neurological or muscular symptoms associated with the mental retardation? For example, does this individual have seizures, problems with coordination and/or walking, poor muscle tone (hypotonia), or muscle weakness?" Congenital myotonic dystrophy is associated with hypotonia and mental retardation with a family history of muscle weakness. Individuals with tuberous sclerosis may have a seizure disorder, mental retardation, hypopigmented spots, and periungual fibromas of the nails. Epilepsy with progressive muscle weakness is a common feature of the mitochondrial encephalopathies.

4.6 AUTISM

Autism is one of the most common developmental disorders. Estimates of the occurrence rate of autism vary from 4.8/10,000 to as high as 1/1000, with males being more commonly affected than females (Wing, 1993; Bryson, 1996). The diagnosis is usually made in the first three years of life, though development in the first year may appear normal (Simonoff and Rutter, 1996). Characteristic features include impairments in processing social and emotional information, language abnormalities (30% have no speech), and repetitive or steroryped behaviors. Mental retardation (IQ below 70) is seen in about 75% of autistic individuals. Their strengths are usually in visuospatial skills, with larger deficits in verbal, abstraction, and conceptualization skills (see reviews in Bryson, 1996; and Simonoff and Rutter, 1997).

Autism has a heterogeneous etiology. A chromosome anomaly should be considered in any individual with autism, particularly if the individual has any minor physical anomalies (see Table 4.3). Chromosome duplications at 15q (the Prader–Willi/Angelman syndrome critical region) have been reported, along with other chromosome anomalies (Cook et al., 1998). The most common inherited syndromes associated with autism include (Simonoff and Rutter, 1997):

- Fragile X syndrome, which affects between 3 and 5% of autisitic individuals, and is inherited in an X-linked pattern
- Tuberous sclerosis complex, an autosomal dominant condition affecting 3–4% of individuals with autism
- Rett syndrome (an X-linked condition with lethality in males) is often confused with autism
- Untreated phenylketonuria

TABLE 4.13 Medical-Family History Questions for Autism

- At what age were the problems with language/socialization/behavior noted?
- Do you know the individual's IQ? (obtain records)
- Does the individual or any family members have:
    A large head?
    Any unusual facial characteristics?
    Any minor physical anomalies?
    A history of seizures?
    Any unusual birthmarks or skin problems?
    Any other medical prblems?
- What type of diagnostic testing has been done?
    Has the individual had a routine karyotype and/or fragile X DNA studies? (obtain actual results)
- Were there any complications with the pregnancy or birth of the child?
- Is there a family history of:
    Miscarriages?
    Mental retardation, learning disabilities, or autism?
    Behavioral problems?
- Are the parents related as blood relatives?

Other features associated with autism include a head size above that of the 97th percentile, epilepsy (affecting about 25%), a history of minor obstetric complications (unexplained by environmental risk factors), and minor congenital anomalies particularly involving the external ear (Rodier et al., 1997; Rutter et al., 1994; Simonoff and Rutter, 1997).

Autistic disorder is considered to have a polygenic/multifactorial etiology. The chance that parents of a child with autism will have another affected child is 3–7% (unless a genetic syndrome is the cause) (Simonoff and Rutter, 1997). The siblings of an individual with autism are also at slightly increased risk to have behavioral problems, as well as subtle deficits in speech, language, and social functioning (Simonoff and Rutter, 1997). The medical-family history questions related to autism are reviewed in Table 4.13.

4.7 NEUROLOGICAL AND NEUROMUSCULAR DISORDERS

Molecular diagnosis is creating an upheaval in the classification systems of genetic neurological diseases. The spinocerebellar ataxias are now classified by at least seven subtypes depending on the molecular etiology. The nomenclature flip-flops back and forth between the hereditary motor sensory neuropathies (HMSN) and the subtypes of Charcot–Marie–Tooth (CMT) as molecular diagnosis refines the phenotypes. Many of the forms of muscular dystrophy can now be distinguished by molecular testing. This flurry of molecular advances is not only recasting the stage of how we think about neurological disorders; but molecular genetic blood tests may also save a person from invasive procedures such as muscle or nerve biopsies. The family-medical history is often the first step in decision-making for a diagnostic evaluation. Coupled with the findings from the patient's neurological exam, the medical-family history guides the clinician in choosing from the myriad of diagnostic tools available for neurological diagnosis. For references surveying the ever-changing field of neurogenetics see Emery (1998), Baraitser (1997), and the London Dysmorphology Database (refer to Appendix A.5: The Genetics Library).

Many hereditary neurological disorders are clinically complex because the nervous system is intimately intertwined with other organ systems. Table 4.14 outlines a broad approach to taking a medical-family history for a neurological condition. This section is followed by more specific guidelines for directed medical-family histories for seizures (Table 4.15), dementia (Table 4.17), and mental illness (Table 4.18). Several hereditary conditions with neurological impairment also include hearing loss (see Section 4.3) and/or visual impairment (see Section 4.4). Cardiomyopathies are common in the muscular dystrophies (see Section 4.11). Inherited metabolic disorders are a frequent inherited cause of progressive neurological conditions, particularly in children. Table 4.11 reviews some of the medical-family history indicators of an inborn error of metabolism.

TABLE 4.14   Medical-Family History Questions for Neurological Disorders[a]

- Describe the problems. Are they with strength? With sensation? With weakness? With coordination? With intellect?
- What studies have been done (e.g., nerve biopsy, muscle biopsy, nerve conduction studies, spinal taps; imaging of the brain and/or spinal cord by MRI, PET, or CT scans; metabolic testing such as organic and/or amino acids, molecular testing)?
- What parts of the body are affected? For example, are there problems with weakness in the following:

   Hands: Does the person drop things, or have trouble holding a pen/pencil?

   Feet: Does the person trip frequently, or have trouble lifting his or her feet such that they make a "slapping sound" when walking?

   Are the feet unusually shaped? For example, does anyone have very high arches, claw or hammer toes? (common in CMT/HMSN)

   Face: Are there problems with smiling, whistling, using a straw? (common in FSHMD and MMD)

   Arms: Does the person have trouble lifting things?

   Does the person have problems combing his/her hair?

   Legs: Do you notice anything unusual about the shape of the legs? (For example, unusually   large calves are seen in Duchenne–Becker muscular dystrophy; thin calves are   seen in the hereditary neuropathies)
- At what age did these problems begin?
- At what age did the individual begin walking? (normal is between 10 and 15 months)
- Was the individual ever able to run?
- Did (does) he or she participate in sports? Explain
- Are the problems getting worse over time or are they stable? If worse, over what period of time? (e.g., 5 years ago, past 5 months)
- Is this person able to walk on his or her own or does he or she require assistance (e.g., cane, wheelchair)?
- Is there anything unusual about the way this person looks compared to other family members? If yes, explain
- Are there *other neurological disorders* in this individual or in other family members, such as:

   Seizures? (see Section 4.8)

   Dysarthria (slurred speech)? (common in many of these disorders but particularly the hereditary ataxias)

   Mental retardation or learning disabilties? (see Section 4.5)

   Problems with thinking or judgment? (note age at onset)

   Problems with memory? (note age at onset)

   Uncontrolled movements? (common in Huntington disease)

   Gait disturbances?

   Spastic movements?

   Stiff movements?

   Depression or mental illness? (see Section 4.10)
- Does this person or do other family members have a problem with alcohol abuse or chemical dependency?
- Does this person, or other family members, have other diseases or medical conditions? Focus on:

   Hearing loss? Note age at onset (common in NF2, several of the cerebellar ataxias, mitochondrial myopathies, associated with some forms of HMSN/CMT) (see Section 4.3)

   Visual impairment? Note age at onset (Visual disturbances are frequently associated with neurological disorders, particularly retinopathies with or without mental retardation. Early onset cataracts are common in MMD) (see Section 4.4)

(continued)

TABLE 4.14 (continued)

Skeletal anomalies, including problems with posture?
Short stature (see Section 4.14)
Heart disease? (particularly myopathies and cardiac conduction defects) (see Section 4.11)
Diabetes? (see Section 4.15)
Thyroid disease?
Any unusual birthmarks or pigmentary changes? (common in tuberous sclerosis, NF, cerebrotendinous xanthomatosis, and some of the rarer cerebellar ataxias)
Infertility? (Can be seen in men with late-onset adrenoleukodystrophy, spinobulbar muscular atrophy, and myotonic muscular dystrophy)
Cancer? (An occult carcinoma may cause symptoms of an acquired ataxia)
• What is the family's ethnic background/country of origin? (For some neurological conditions there is a founder effect such that certain gene alterations are easier to identify in certain groups, or the disorder may occur more frequently in individuals of certain ancestries)
• Are the parents of the individual related as cousins or more closely related?

[a]Abbreviations: CMT = Charcot–Marie–Tooth disease; FSHMD = fascioscapulohumeral muscular dystrophy; HMSN = hereditary motor-sensory neuropathies; MMD = myotonic muscular dystrophy; NF = neurofibromatosis.

4.8 SEIZURES

Epilepsy is a group of disorders with many causes. Approximately 0.5–1.0% of the general population has recurrent seizures (Bird, 1992). By definition, epilepsy is a disorder of the brain, characterized by recurrent, unprovoked, epileptic seizures. An epileptic seizure is a transient episode of cortical neuronal activity manifesting as a motor, sensory, autonomic, cognitive, or psychic disturbance (Elmslie and Gardiner,1997). Myoclonic epilepsy is a common feature of inborn errors of metabolism and mitochondrial disorders (features of mitochondrial disorders are summarized in Table 2.5). Acquired epilepsy can result from any brain injury such as head trauma, meningitis or encephalitis, asphyxia (prenatal or postnatal), and hypoxia–ischemia from cerebrovascular disease.

Epilepsy may occur in isolation or as part of a syndrome (single gene, chromosomal, or mitochondrial). More than 200 inherited syndromes are associated with seizure disorders (Elmslie and Gardiner, 1997). A general epilepsy syndrome may be associated with several different varieties of seizures. For example, generalized tonic–clonic, myoclonic, and absence seizures may occur in juvenile myoclonic epilepsy. A clear genetic cause of epilepsy is identified in approximately 20% of patients (Elmslie and Gardiner, 1997). Generalized idiopathic epilepsy is common, affecting approximately 1/200 individuals (Baraitser, 1997). A sibling or child of an individual with epilepsy has a 2–10% risk to develop a seizure disorder (Bird, 1992). The risk of occurrence is higher in the children of mothers with epilepsy, when compared to the offspring of fathers with a seizure disorder.

Questions to ask for a family history of seizures are listed in Table 4.15. Seizures are a presenting sign, or an evolving feature, of many of the inborn errors of metab-

TABLE 4.15 Medical-Family History Questions for a Seizure Disorder[a]

- Do you know the type of seizures? (partial simple, partial complex, generalized absence, generalized tonic–clonic)
- Were the seizures single or repeated?
- Did the seizure occur with an illness or fever?
- At what age (infancy, childhood, as an adult) did the seizures begin?
- Did the individual with seizures have any type of brain trauma or infection?
- What medications does the individual with seizures take?
- Did the mother of the person with seizures have any infections in pregnancy? (can be seen in fetal toxoplasmosis, rubella, herpes, and CMV)
- Does any other family member have seizures? Who?

- Does the person with seizures or any family members have:
  Unusual facial features?
  > Coarsening of facial features (with MR) can be seen in storage diseases (AR or XL)
  > Dysmorphic facial features (with MR) seen in several chromosome anomalies
  > Large head, protruding jaw and ears (with MR) characteristic of fragile X syndrome (XL—trinucleotide repeat)

  Unusual facial acne? (angiofibromas) are characteristic of tuberous sclerosis complex (TSC) (AD with variable expressivity)
  Impaired hearing? (see Section 4.3)
  Problems with vision? (see Section 4.4)
  Unusual skin findings?
  > White (ashleaf) spots (common in TSC)
  > Brown (café au lait) spots, common in neurofibromatosis 1 (NF1) (AD with variable expressivity)
  > Swirls of patchy hypopigmentation (with MR), characteristic of hypomelanosis of Ito (Chromosomal mosaicism/unknown)
  > Marbled, swirly patches of skin, characteristic of incontinentia pigmenti (XL dominant)
  > Red/purple "port wine" stains (nevus flammeus) seen in Sturge–Weber syndrome (sporadic)
  > Yellow/orange/tan nevi seen in sebaceous nevus sequence (?sporadic)
  > Fatty benign tumors (lipomas)

  Unusual lumps or growths?
  > Lumps (neurofibromas in NF1; angiofibromas in TSC)
  > Growths under nails (periungual fibromas) pathognomonic for TSC

  Mental retardation or learning disabilities? (see Section 4.5)
  > (can be seen with NF1, TSC, fragile X syndrome, maternal teratogens, chromosome anomalies, and inborn errors of metabolism including storage disorders)

  Problems with walking (gait disturbance)? Note age at onset (see Section 4.7)
  > (Can be seen with several of the hereditary ataxias, mitochondrial myopathies, and inborn errors of metabolism)

  Difficulty with coordination?
  Muscle weakness?
  Problems with behavior, thinking, or judgment? (see Table 4.18 and Section 4.10)

- Are the parents of the individual with seizures blood relatives; for example, are they cousins?

---

[a]Abbreviations: MR = mental retardation; NF1 = neurofibromatosis 1; TSC = tuberous sclerosis complex; AD = autosomal dominant; AR = autosomal recessive; XL = X-linked.
Sources: Baraitser, 1997; Bird, 1992; Sybert, 1997.

olism (particularly the storage disorders). Some of the common symptoms of inborn errors of metabolism are listed in Table 4.11. It is important to obtain documentation of any medical evaluations such as EEGs (electroencephalograms), brain imaging studies (CT, MRI), ophthalmologic testing, metabolic testing (plasma amino acids, urine organic acids), and pathology reports from biopsies of skin lesions. Several anticonvulsant agents are toxic to the fetus during pregnancy (see Table 3.2). Seizure control and the potential teratogenic effects of medication on a developing fetus are important considerations in managing the pregnancy of a woman with a seizure disorder and should be discussed in genetic counseling.

4.9 DEMENTIA

> From past generations we receive a few strands of DNA, sometimes a heritage, a memory of one sort or another.
>
> —Daniel A. Pollen (1993)

For individuals older than 90, the prevalence of dementia is estimated to be approximately 43% of the population (Heston, 1992). The overall lifetime risk to develop Alzheimer disease is 5% (Baraitser, 1997). As defined by the Royal College of Physicians, dementia is "the global impairment of higher cortical functions including learned perceptuomotor skills, the correct use of social skills, and control of emotional reactions in the absence of gross clouding of consciousness. The condition is often irreversible and progressive" (Roses and Pericak-Vance, 1997). A neuropathological diagnosis is required to determine the type of dementia. If your patient has a living first-degree relative with dementia, encourage your patient to discuss the delicate subject of neuropathology with his or her family members. For deceased family members, it is essential to obtain neuropathology records to provide accurate genetic assessment for other family members. On several occasions I have been involved with a patient evaluation in which we actually obtained ancient neuropathology slides. These slides were re-interpreted by a neuropathologist, which resulted in a new diagnosis and an alteration in the genetic counseling.

Most dementia is not inherited. Noninherited causes of dementia include acquired immunodeficiency syndrome, syphilis, central nervous system infections, vascular disease (e.g. strokes), metabolic or nutritional deficiencies (e.g., thyroid and B_{12} deficiency), and drug toxicity (Roses and Pericak-Vance, 1997).

Huntington disease should be considered in any adult with a movement disorder, incoordination, and problems with thinking and judgment. It is inherited as an autosomal dominant trait, so usually there is a family history of the condition. Because this is a trinucleotide repeat disorder (see Chapter 3), an individual who has an apparent new mutation most likely has a parent with a CAG repeat expansion in the intermediate range (ACMG/ASHG, 1998).

Familial Alzheimer disease (FAD), a rare cause of dementia, has been mapped to several different chromosomes. The primary family history feature that suggests FAD is dementia and memory loss of early onset (prior to age 55 years), that is inherited in an autosomal dominant pattern. Other rare causes of Alzheimer-like de-

TABLE 4.16 Inherited Disorders Associated with Adult-Onset Dementia

Disorder	Inheritance Pattern	Other Clinical Features
CADASIL[a]	AD	Relapsing strokes, seizures, migraines, motor disabilities, mood swings/depression
Choreoacanthocytosis	AD	Chorea, acanthocytes (red-cell anomaly), dystonia
Creutzfeldt-Jakob disease	Sporadic, AD	Ataxia, jerky trembling movements (usually transmitted as a sporadic prion disease)
DRPLA[b]	AD	Seizures, choreoathetosis
Gerstmann–Straussler disease	AD	Cerebellar ataxia
Gliosis, familial subcortical	?AR	Neuropathological distinctions from familial Alzheimer disease
Frontal lobe dementia	?AD	Neuropathological distinctions from familial Alzheimer disease (one type, FTDP-17[c] is AD)
Hallervorden–Spatz disease	AR	Retinitis pigmentosa, gait abnormalities, dystonia, chorea, seizures
Huntington disease	AD	Chorea, incoordination
Kearns-Sayres syndrome	MT	Cerebellar ataxia, ophthalmoplegia, retinal degeneration, seizures, sensorineural deafness, short stature, cardiac conduction defects
Lewy body dementia	Sporadic, AD	Dysphasia, Parkinsonism
MELAS[d]	MT	Seizures, sensorineural deafness, cortical blindness, renal anomalies, short stature, headaches, diabetes
MERRF[e]	MT	Cerebellar ataxia, myoclonus, seizures, sensorineural deafness, short stature
Pick disease	sporadic, AD	Neuropathological distinctions from familial Alzheimer disease
Spinocerebellar ataxia type 2	AD	Cerebellar ataxia, dysarthria, optic atrophy

[a]Cerebral autosomal dominant arteriopathy with subcortical infarcts and leukoencepahlopathy.
[b]Dentatorubro-pallidoluysian atrophy.
[c]Frontotemporal dementia with Parkinsonism—chromosome 17 linked.
[d]Mitochondrial encephalomyopathy, lactic acidosis and stroke-like episodes.
[e]Myoclonic epilepsy and ragged-red fibers.
Sources: Clarke, 1996; OMIM, 1998; Roses and Pericak-Vance, 1997; Saudubray and Charpentier, 1995.

mentia (see Table 4.16) include Pick disease, frontal lobe dementia, and Lewy body disease (all usually sporadic but sometimes autosomal dominant), and subcortical gliosis (autosomal recessive) (OMIM, 1998; Roses and Pericak-Vance, 1997). These conditions can be distinguished from FAD only by neuropathological distinctions.

There are several uncommon metabolic disorders (all inherited in an autosomal recessive pattern) associated with the development of dementia in childhood (before age 15 years) (adapted from Saudubray and Charpentier, 1995):

- Ceroid lipofuscinosis
- Gaucher disease III (juvenile or Norrbottnian type)
- Lafora disease
- Niemann–Pick type C
- Proprionic acidemia
- Sandhoff disease
- Sialidosis
- Late-onset Tay–Sachs disease (GM2 gangliosidosis)

Refer to Table 4.11 for the medical-family history features suggestive of inborn errors of metabolism. Many of the conditions that are associated with childhood or adult-onset dementia are also seen in individuals that have behavioral disorders or mental illness as a frequent presenting manifestation of the disease (see Table 4.18). Several of the mitochondrial myopathies (Kearns–Sayres syndrome, MERRF, and MELAS) may also present with dementia in childhood or as an adult (Clarke, 1996).

The medical-family history questions for sorting out a hereditary etiology for dementia are reviewed in Table 4.17.

TABLE 4.17 Medical-Family History Questions for Dementia

- At what age did your family member(s) develop dementia? (onset of dementia before age 60 is more likely to have a hereditary component)
- If deceased, was a brain autopsy performed? (obtain pathology reports)
- Have any brain imaging studies been done, such as an MRI or CT scan? (obtain reports)
- Does/do the person(s) with dementia drink alcohol or use street drugs? (note type of substance, how much, and for how long)
- Does the affected individual or anyone in the family have:
    Problems with speech? Describe and note age at onset
    Difficulty with hearing? Note age at onset (see Section 4.3)
    Problems with vision? Note age at onset (see Section 4.4)
    Problems with coordination or walking? Note age at onset
    Muscle weakness? If so, was a muscle biopsy performed?
    A history of strokes or stroke-like episodes? Note age at onset
    Uncontrolled movements (chorea)? Note age at onset
    A seizure disorder? Note age at onset, and type if known (see Section 4.8)

4.10 MENTAL ILLNESS

Individuals with mental illness in the family are often profoundly concerned about their own chances of developing a mental disorder or of having affected children. These fears are partly because of the significant aura of stigmatization and shame that is traditionally associated with a diagnosis of mental illness (Kinney, 1997). Providing genetic risk assessment for these individuals is frustrating, mainly because the definitions of mental illness rest on shifting territory. The studies from

TABLE 4.18   Genetic Disorders That May Present with Psychiatric or Severe Behavioral Abnormalities[a]

Condition	Age of Onset of Mental Illness	Inheritance
Adrenoleukodystrophy/adrenal myeloneuropathy	Childhood–young adults	XL
CADASIL	Young adults	AD
Cerebrotendinous xanthomatosis[b]	Teens–adulthood	AR
DRPLA	Adulthood	AD
Fragile X syndrome[b]	Variable	XL
FTDP-17	Adulthood	AD
GM2 gangliosidosis (late-onset Tay–Sachs)	Teens–adulthood	AR
Hartnup disorder	Variable	AR
Homocystinuria[b]	Variable	AR
Huntington disease	Adult	AD
Juvenile Huntington disease	5–15 years	AD (usually father is affected)
Krabbe disease[b]	5–15 years	AR
Lafora disease	5–15 years	AR
Leigh syndrome	5–15 years	MT, AR
Metachromatic leukodystrophy, late-onset	20+ years	AR
Methylene tetrahydrofolate reductase deficiency	Variable	AR
Neuronal ceroid lipofuscinosis (Kufs disease)	Variable	AR, ?AD
Niemann–Pick Type C	Teens–adulthood	AR
Ornithine transcarbamylase deficiency (late onset)	Variable	XL
Phenylketonuria (poor dietary control)	Adults	AR
Pick disease	Teens–adult	AD
Porphyrias	Teens–adult	
Acute intermittent porphyria		AD
Copoporphyria		AD
Porphyria variegata		AD
Sanfilippo syndrome[b]	Childhood	AR
Velocardiofacial syndrome[b]	Teens–adult	AD
Wilson disease	Variable	AR

[a]Abbreviations: AD = autosomal dominant, AR = autosomal recessive, XL = X-linked, MT = mitochondrial, CADASIL = cerebral autosomal dominant arteriopathy with subcortical infaracts and leukoencephalopathy, DRPLA = dentatorubro-pallidoluysian atrophy, FTDP-17 = frontotemporal dementia with Parkinsonism—chromosome 17 linked
[b]Associated with learning disabilities.
Sources: Baraitser, 1997; Carlson et al., 1997; Clarke, 1996; Hanson and Gottesman, 1992; Saudubray and Charpentier, 1995; Thomas Bird, personal communication.

which empirical risk figures are drawn depend on the criteria chosen for diagnosis of the mental illness; but the classifications of mental illness have changed over time. For example, some investigators use a broad definition of manic depressive illness, others use more specific diagnoses such as bipolar disorder type I and bipolar disorder type II (MacKinnon et al., 1997). To confuse nosology further, schizophrenia is distinct from manic depressive disorders, yet mood disorders can have psychotic features. Additional classification dilemmas arise when confronted with the milder clinical spectrum of mood disorders such as hypomania without major depression, dysthymia, and seasonal depression disorders (cyclothymia).

TABLE 4.19   Family Medical-History Queries for Mental Illness

- Formal psychiatric diagnosis (try to obtain medical records)
- Age at onset of mental illness
- Medications
- Does the person have a history of drug or alcohol abuse?
- Does the person have other medical problems? In particular is there a history of:
  Learning disabilities or mental retardation? If yes, see Section 4.5.
  Any unusual movements? (e.g., Huntington disease, Wilson disease, Hallervorden–
    Spatz)
  Seizures? If yes, see Section 4.8
  Problems with coordination?
  Sun sensitivity (photosensitivity)? (porphyria, Hartnup disorder)
  Any unusual lumps? (could be xanthomas)
  Chronic diarrhea? (Hartnup disorder, Sanfilippo syndrome)
  Acute abdominal pain? (porphyrias)
- Do any family members have mental illness or other medical problems (as above)?
- Have any family members attempted or committed suicide?
- Are the parents of the individual blood relatives?

The prevalence of schizophrenia differs around the world and may reflect variation in culture, gene pools, and diagnostic practice (Kinney, 1997). The overall lifetime prevalence is usually quoted as between 0.1 and 1% (Kinney, 1997). There are
several known genetic disorders to consider when there is a family history of schizophrenic-like symptoms (see Table 4.18). Two metabolic disorders that are treatable
include Wilson disease and acute intermittent porphyria. Hartnup disorder is an autosomal recessive inborn error of metabolism (characterized by light-sensitive skin
changes similar to the rash of pellagra), and associated with cerebellar ataxia and
episodic psychotic features. Expression seems to be associated with dietary factors
and it is treatable with oral nicotinamide (Sybert, 1997). Nonhereditary causes of
schizophrenic-like disorders include brain injury or malformation (e.g., physical
trauma, brain tumor, embolism, or ischemia), viral encephalitis, syphilis, chronic alcoholism, drug abuse (particularly cocaine, crack, LSD, PCP, or amphetamines),
and metabolic/systemic disease (e.g., hypoglycemia, vitamin B_{12} deficiency, systemic lupus erythematosus, uremic syndrome, hepatic encephalopathy, pellagra)
(Hanson and Gottesman, 1992; Kinney, 1997).

Obtaining medical-family history information for a psychiatric illness can be
challenging. The report of which family members are affected with a psychiatric
disorder may differ depending on which relative is interviewed (Kendler, 1997). A
study of twins, one of whom had a history of major depression and the other did
not, suggested that the twin with major depression was more likely to report depression in their mother than the twin without major depression (Kendler et al., 1991).
Family members may be protective of this private information because of fears of
ostracism or feelings of shame. The parents of a person with mental illness may fear
their parenting styles caused their child's problems; probing questions may exacer-
bate their feelings of guilt. A parent with profound mental illness may be a poor historian. Though it is optimal to review medical records on affected family members,

psychiatric records are often difficult to obtain on both living and deceased individuals, despite written permission from the affected individual or next-of-kin. Table 4.19 reviews the family-medical history questions for mental illness.

4.11 DISORDERS INVOLVING THE CARDIAC SYSTEM

In the past 10 years, molecular genetic techniques have redefined the classification and methods of evaluating cardiac dysfunction. Heart disease can be broadly separated into the following categories (Coonar and McKeena, 1997; Schievink, 1998):

- **Cardiomyopathies (disease of the heart muscle):**

  Hypertrophic (HCM). At least four autosomal dominant genes have been identified: *beta-cardiac myosin, troponin T, alpha-tropomyosin,* and *myosin-binding protein C,* which account for at most 50% of HCM;

  Dilated (DCM). At least 20–25% are suspected to be inherited, most of which are autosomal dominant or X-linked;

  Arrhythmogenic right ventricular (ARVC). These are usually autosomal dominant or autosomal recessive;

  Restrictive (RCM). It is debatable whether or not this truly represents a distinct category of cardiomyopathy, and how RCM is distinguished from endocardial fibroelastosis is unclear.

- **Structural cardiovascular anomalies:**

  Congenital heart defects (e.g., velocardiofacial/DiGeorge syndrome, Holt–Oram syndrome);

  Aneurysms. Marfan syndrome, polycystic kidney disease, vascular type (IV) Ehlers–Danlos syndrome (all autosomal dominant), and alpha 1-antitrypsin deficiency (autosomal recessive), should be considered if there is a history of familial aneurysms;

  Valve defects (such as mitral valve prolapse).

- *Cardiac conduction defects* (diseases of heart rhythm) such as primary long QT syndrome. Multiple loci have been identified, including three autosomal dominant genes associated with the Romano–Ward phenotype, and the autosomal recessive Jervell–Lange–Nielsen syndrome associated with deafness.

- *Dyslipoproteinemias* are associated with abnormalities in the metabolism of plasma lipoproteins and their associated apoproteins, which in turn significantly increase the risk for atherosclerosis and coronary artery disease. They are among the most common genetic disorders in Westernized countries, and they are inherited in an autosomal dominant pattern.

The person you are obtaining a family history from is unlikely to separate a relative's heart disease into distinct categories as outlined above. Obtaining medical records such as echocardiograms (an ultrasound of the heart), electrocardiogram reports (cardiac rhythm studies), studies of vascular function, surgical reports, and pathology from surgical specimens, cardiac and muscle biopsies, plasma lipoprotein and apoprotein studies, creatine kinase levels, molecular analysis, and autopsy reports is essential for genetic diagnosis and risk assessment.

The important aspects to document in the medical-family history with regard to heart disease are outlined in Table 4.20. When there is a family history of a congen-

---

TABLE 4.20   Medical-Family History Questions for Cardiac Disease

Information on Person with Cardiac Disease

- At what age was the heart disease diagnosed? Cardiomyopathies in an infant are more likely to have a mitochondrial, autosomal recessive (AR), or X-linked (XL) etiology. Autosomal dominant (AD) inheritance is more common with later age of onset cardiomyopathies.
- Is the person living or deceased?
  If deceased, was an autopsy done? (obtain autopsy report)
- Was the heart disease of sudden onset? Did the person know he or she had heart disease for a long time?
- Did (does) the person have a history of any chronic infections or autoimmune disease?
- Did (does) the person have a history of high blood pressure?
- Did (does) the person use alcohol? Tobacco? How heavily?
- Do you know what medications the person takes/took?
- What surgeries (cardiovascular or otherwise) have been performed? (obtain surgical and pathology reports)
- Do you know what medical/diagnostic studies have been done? (obtain reports)
- Does this person have other medical problems? Explain.
- Were there any complications after the birth of this individual, such as floppiness (hypotonia)?

Information on Person with Cardiovascular Disease and Other Family Members

- Any history of strokes? If yes, what was the age at onset?
- Any history of sudden death? If yes, what was the age at death? (obtain pathology reports)
- Is there a history of neuromuscular disease? Cardiomyopathy is secondary to several neuromuscular disorders such as myotonic muscular dystrophy (AD), Friedreich ataxia (AR), Duchenne–Becker and Emery–Dreifuss muscular dystrophies (both XL), the limb-girdle muscular dystrophies, and mitochondrial disorders such as Kearns–Sayre syndrome, MELAS, and MERRF.
- Any history of hearing loss? Jervell–Lange–Nielsen syndrome (AR) and multiple lentigines syndrome (AD) are associated with hearing loss.
- Any unusual skin findings? Xanthomas are seen in many of the dyslipoproteinemias; restrictive cardiomyopathy and angiokeratomas in Fabry disease (XL); restrictive cardiomyopathy and "bronze" skin in hemochromatosis (AR); fragile, hyperelastic skin in vascular Ehlers–Danlos (type IV) (AD); peau d'orange skin in pseudoxanthoma elasticum (AD, AR).
- Anyone unusually tall or short? Routinely obtain parental and sibling heights. Marfan syndrome (AD) and homocystinuria (AR) are associated with tall stature. Turner syndrome (CH) and Noonan syndrome (AD) are associated with short stature.
- Any history of unusual bruising? Can be seen in vascular Ehlers–Danlos (type IV) (AD).

(continued)

TABLE 4.20   *(continued)*

- Anyone with problems with healing? Can be seen in vascular Ehlers–Danlos (type IV) (AD).
- Any history of loose joints or hyperextensibility? Can be seen in connective tissue disorders such as vascular Ehlers–Danlos (type IV) (AD) and Marfan syndrome (AD).
- Is there a history of scoliosis (curvature of the spine)? Can be seen in connective tissue disorders and neuromuscular diseases.
- Is there anything unusual about the way the person looks? Dilated cardiomyopathy is associated with Noonan syndrome.
- Is there anyone in the family with early frontal balding? Can be seen in myotonic muscular dystrophy.
- Is there a family history of learning disabilities or mental retardation? Myotonic dystrophy, Noonan syndrome, and homocystinuria are associated with learning disabilities.
- Do any family members have cataracts? (see Table 4.10)
- Do any family members have a seizure disorder? (see Section 4.8)
- Is there a history of spontaneous pneumothorax? Can be seen in Marfan syndrome.
- Is there any history of chronic disease in this person or other family members? Note in particular a history of diabetes, kidney disease, liver disease, and thyroid disease.
- Is there a family history of pregnancy loss, stillborns, or early childhood deaths?
- Are the parents related as blood relatives?

Sources: Clarke, 1996; Coonar and McKeena, 1997.

ital heart defect, the family history queries are similar as for other birth defects, as I have outlined in Section 4.2 and Table 4.4. Cardiomyopathies that present before the age of 4 years are often due to mitochondrial disorders or inborn errors of metabolism (particularly storage disorders), which are inherited in an autosomal recessive or X-linked pattern (Clarke, 1996). Family history features suggestive of a mitochondrial disorder or inborn errors of metabolism are reviewed in Tables 2.5 and 2.6, and 4.11, respectively. For an illuminating review on the complicated subject of familial cardiomyopathy see Coonar and McKeena (1997). Clarke (1996) provides a concise discussion of several of the inherited metabolic disorders in which cardomyopathies are a prominent feature.

4.12 CHRONIC RESPIRATORY DISEASE

Hereditary influences on common respiratory conditions (such as asthma) are just beginning to be elucidated. It is most likely that several genes are involved, with gene expression influenced by environmental exposures to allergens, air pollutants, and smoking. The major single gene contributors to respiratory disease are cystic fibrosis and alpha-1-antitrypsin deficiency. Individuals with Young syndrome or Kartagener syndrome may have chronic sinopulmonary infections. Cystic fibrosis should also be considered in individuals who appear to have Young syndrome or Kartagener syndrome. All four conditions are autosomal recessive. The carrier frequency of cystic fibrosis is common enough in some ethnic populations that it is not unusual to see cystic fibrosis occur in more distantly related family members (for example, related as a cousin, niece, or nephew to a person with cystic fibrosis). An

TABLE 4.21   **Medical-Family History Questions for Chronic Respiratory Disease**

- Has the individual always had respiratory problems? If not, at what age did the problems begin?
- Does this person smoke cigarettes, or has he or she smoked cigarettes in the past? How many packs per day, and for how long?
- What is this person's occupation? (Could the lung disease be related to occupational exposure?)
- What studies have been done? Obtain medical records including:
  Chest x-rays/lung imaging studies
  Pulmonary function studies
  Sweat chloride studies (for CF[a] diagnosis)
  DNA testing (obtain the actual lab results, especially for CF because laboratories use different mutation panels)
  Measurement of serum concentrations of alpha-1-antitrypsin
- What types of medical interventions have been done? Has the individual had any hospitalizations? Any surgeries?
- Does the individual or any family member have a history of:
  Chronic sinusitis?
  Chronic infections?
  Nasal polyps? (can be seen in CF, Young syndrome, and Kartagener syndrome)
  Liver disease?
    Cirrhosis of the liver (can be seen in alpha-1-antitrypsin deficiency)
  Pancreatic disease?
  Gastrointestinal disease?
- Does the person have a history of fatty, foul-smelling stools? (seen in CF)
- Has this person had problems conceiving a pregnancy? (can be seen in CF, Young syndrome, and Kartagener syndrome)
- What is the person's ethnic origin?
  Alpha-1-antitrypsin deficiency is rare in individuals of Asian or African American ancestry
  The frequency of CF mutations varies widely based on ethnicity. Knowing the family ancestry can help the clinician interpret DNA testing
- Are the parents related as cousins or more closely related?

[a]CF = cystic fibrosis.

approach to directed medical-family history queries for chronic respiratory disease is shown in Table 4.21.

4.13 RENAL DISORDERS

Hereditary renal disorders can be divided into six general categories (Morgan, 1998):

1. *Malformations of the kidney and urinary tract.* There are several hundred syndromes and single gene disorders involving congenital structural disorders of the kidney, urinary tract, and valves (Van Allen, 1997). Approximately 35% of individuals with chromosomal disorders have renal anomalies (Van Allen, 1997). Teratogens known to affect the development of the kidney and ureters include alcohol, alkylating agents, angiotensin-converting enzyme inhibitors,

cocaine, maternal diabetes, rubella, thalidomide, trimethadione, and vitamin A derivatives (Van Allen, 1997).

2. *Cystic diseases of the kidney.* Kidney cysts (often congenital) are a component of several hereditary syndromes. Multiple renal cysts are associated with single gene disorders, chromosome anomalies, maternal alcohol use, uncontrolled maternal diabetes, and fetal rubella. In adults, autosomal dominant polycystic disease, tuberous sclerosis complex (AD), and von Hippel–Lindau syndrome (AD) should be considered.

3. *Glomerular disorders* such as:

    Congenital nephrosis (nephrotic syndrome) (AR)

    Renal amyloidosis (AD) (see below)

    Hereditary nephritis. The most common cause of inherited nephritis is Alport syndrome (a heterogeneous group of disorders, characterized by sensorineural hearing loss with renal disease, that are inherited in AD, AR, and XL patterns).

    Nail-patella syndrome (onycho-osteodysplasia) (AD)

    Uremic syndromes

4. *Tubular disorders* such as:

    Nephrogenic diabetes insipidus (NDI) (usually X-linked with females often being symptomatic, rarely autosomal recessive).

    Renal tubular acidosis (RTA) (Clarke, 1996). With the exception of Wilson disease, RTA is rarely the presenting problem in these individuals. Some examples of inborn errors of metabolism with RTA include:

    Carnitine palmitoyl transferase 1 (AR)

    Cystinosis (AR)

    Cytochrome-*c*-oxidase deficiency (congenital lactic acidosis) (AR)

    Galactosemia (AR)

    Hereditary fructose intolerance (AR)

    Hypophosphatemic rickets (XL with expression in females)

    Lowe syndrome (XL)

    Pyruvate carboxylase deficiency (AR)

    Tyrosinemia (hepatorenal) (AR)

    Wilson disease (AR)

5. *Inborn errors of metabolism* including:

    Fabry disease (XL condition resulting in renal failure from glycosphingolipid deposition)

    Glutaric acidemia type II (multiple acyl-CoA-dehydrogenase deficiency)

    Certain hereditary amyloidoses (heterogeneous group of disorders all inherited as autosomal dominants)

    Sickle cell disease (AR)

    Peroxisomal disorders (AR and XL) (e.g., Zellweger syndrome)

6. *Phakomatoses and kidney cancers*

Tuberous sclerosis complex (more than one autosomal dominant locus)

Von Hippel–Lindau syndrome (autosomal dominant with hemangioblas-tomas and renal cell carcinoma)

Wilms' tumor syndromes (heterogeneous)

A general approach to medical-family history queries for renal disorders is shown in Table 4.22.

TABLE 4.22   Medical-Family History Questions for Renal Disorders

---

Prenatal History

Was there anything unusual about the prenatal history of the individual (for example, oligohydramnios)?

Did this person's mother:

- Use alcohol during the pregnancy? If so, when during the pregnancy, how often, and how much?
- Use cocaine during the pregnancy? If so, how often?
- Have diabetes during the pregnancy?
- Take any medications during the pregnancy (specifically vitamin A congeners, trimethadione)?
- Have any infections during pregnancy?
- Have any testing done in the pregnancy such as serum maternal-fetal marker screening or fetal chromosomal studies?

Individual's Medical History

What was the age at onset of the renal disorder?

What studies have been done? (obtain documentation of renal function studies, abdominal imaging studies, biopsies)

Does (did) the individual drink alcohol? How much?

Were there any anomalies noted at birth or shortly thereafter? (e.g., microcephaly, cleft lip/palate, heart defects, neural tube defects, hand and feet anomalies, limb anomalies, skeletal anomalies)

What is this person's occupation? (could this be a toxic exposure, such as lead poisioning leading to renal tubular acidosis?)

Individual and Family History Questions

What is the individual's height? What are the heights of the parents and siblings?

Do any of the family members have high blood pressure?

Have any other family members had testing (such as renal studies on the parents)?

Does this individual, or any family members, have other medical conditions such as:

- Learning disabilities or mental retardation? If yes, see Section 4.5.
- Any unusual birth marks? (tuberous sclerosis, Fabry disease)
- Anything unusual about the shape of the hands or feet, or the nails? (periungual fibromas in tuberous sclerosis, nail hypoplasia in nail-patella syndrome)
- Hearing loss? Commonly seen in many of the inherited renal syndromes. Two of the more common syndromes with hearing loss and renal anomalies are branchio-oto-renal syndrome and Alport syndrome (see Section 4.3)

(continued)

TABLE 4.22 *(continued)*

- Unusually shaped ears?
- Preauricular pits? (e.g., branchio-oto-renal syndrome)
- Ear tags?
- Visual disorders? (see Section 4.4)
    Retinal disease is common (e.g., Bardet–Biedl syndrome)
    Aniridia (absence of the iris is associated with Wilms' tumor syndromes)
    Coloboma (seen in several of the chromosomal syndromes and multiple congenital
        anomaly syndromes)
    Retinal angiomas (von Hippel–Lindau disease)
    Early-onset cataracts (galactosemia, Zellweger syndrome, rhizomelic chondrodysplasia,
        Smith–Lemli–Opitz syndrome, Wilson syndrome, Alport syndrome) (see Tables 4.9 and
        4.10)
    Lenticular opacities (spoke-like) are characteristic of Fabry disease
    Amyloid deposits in some of the hereditary amyloidosis
    Kaiser-Fleischer rings in Wilson disease
    Dark, "cloverleaf" pigmentation at inner margin of irides (nail-patella syndrome)
- Cardiac disease, particularly cardiomyopathies (see Section 4.11)
- Neurological disease (particularly seizures) (see Section 4.7)
    Neuropathy (common in some of the hereditary amyloidosis syndromes)
- Skeletal anomalies? (several skeletal dysplasias are associated with renal disorders) (see
    Section 4.14)
- Genital anomalies or ambiguous genitalia?
- Cancer? (particularly renal cell cancer), which can occur in tuberous sclerosis complex and
    von Hippel–Lindau syndrome) (see Chapter 5)

General Questions

What is the family ethnic background? (This information can be particularly helpful in
    interpreting molecular genetic testing)
Are the parents related as first cousins or closer?

Sources: Clarke, 1996; Morgan and Grunfeld, 1998; Saudubray and Charpentier, 1995; Van Allen, 1997.

4.14 SKELETAL ANOMALIES AND DISORDERS OF SHORT STATURE

"Good things come in small packages."
—My mother

The determinism of what is normal or aberrant when it comes to measuring stature depends on ethnic, familial, and nutritional variables. If, in evaluating a family history, there is concern about a relative with seemingly unusual stature, obtaining growth curves (if available) on the relative is important. Is this person growing along his or her own curve, or does growth seem to have reached a plateau? Documenting parental, grandparental, and sibling heights is also useful. Obtaining the radiographic reports and films, including the bone age, is imperative; the radiographic findings are usually essential for making a diagnosis. Excellent reviews of the radiographic findings in skeletal dysplasias can be found in Taybi and Lachman (1996).

For individuals with short stature, the first step is determining whether or not the individual has proportionate or disproportionate short stature. Persons with disproportionate short stature usually have an inherited skeletal dysplasia or metabolic bone disease. As shown in Table 4.23, individuals with proportionate short stature may have a more generalized disorder attributed to factors such as malnutrition,

TABLE 4.23   Common Causes of Proportionate Short Stature[a]

Prenatal Onset (Intrauterine Growth Retardation or IUGR)

Familial short stature
Constriction of fetal movement (i.e., from lack of amniotic fluid, multiple gestations, uterine anomalies)
Maternal infections (e.g., cytomegalovirus, rubella, varicella, syphilis, toxoplasmosis)
Placental insufficiency
Teratogenic exposures (e.g., alcohol, cocaine, heroin, hydantoin, trimethadione, warfarin)
Chromosomal anomalies (most common are Turner syndrome, trisomies 13 and 18, Down syndrome)
Dysmorphic genetic syndromes

Examples	Inheritance Pattern
Aarskog syndrome	XL
Bloom syndrome	AR
Cockayne syndrome B (II)	AR
Dubowitz syndrome	AR
de Lange syndrome	IM
Fanconi pancytopenia syndrome	AR (multiple syndromes)
Oculomandibulofacial syndrome (Hallerman–Streiff)	?
Noonan syndrome	AD
Opitz syndrome	XL, AD
Rubinstein–Taybi syndrome	16p13.3 del
Smith–Lemli–Opitz syndromes	AR
Williams syndrome	7q11.23 del
Xeroderma pigmentosum	AR, multiple loci

Postnatal Onset

Familial short stature
Chronic malnutrition
Chronic childhood diseases (genetic and nongenetic)
    Cardiac (e.g., congenital heart disease)
    Gastrointestinal
    Pulmonary disease (e.g., cystic fibrosis, alpha-1-antitrypsin)
    Renal
    Hematologic (e.g., hemoglobinopathies)
    Neurological
Chronic infections
Drug effects
Psychosocial/emotional disturbances

[a]Abbreviations: XL = X-linked; AR = autosomal recessive; IM = imprinting; AD = autosomal dominant; del = deletion.
Sources: Graham and Rimoin, 1997; Jones, 1997; Sanders, 1996.

TABLE 4.24   Family-Medical History Questions for Short Stature or Skeletal Dysplasias

Pregnancy History

During her pregnancy, did this individual's mother have:
Diabetes?
High fevers? If yes, at what stage in the pregnancy?
Any infections? Explain
Any prenatal testing, particularly ultrasounds, documenting fetal growth?

General Family History Questions

What are the parental heights and the heights of the siblings? (Ideally the parents should be examined for dysmorphic features and for anomalies particularly in their hands and feet)
What is the family's country of origin?
Are the parents related as first cousins, or more closely related?
Is there a history of miscarriages, stillbirths, or babies who died?

Information on the Individual

Obtain documentation of a full set of skeletal X-rays (including skull, spine, limbs, pelvis, hands, feet, and bone age)
Obtain the childhood growth charts
What is the individual's present height? Document upper to lower segment ratio, sitting height, and arm span
What studies have been done (e.g., cytogenetic, growth hormone assays, thyroid studies, studies for inborn errors of metabolism)?
Is the person with short stature proportionate?
If not, does the person with disproportionate short stature have:
Short limbs?
A short trunk?
Was the short stature evident at birth? Or, did it develop during the first year of life, or later?
Are there any prenatal ultrasounds documenting growth abnormalities?

Does the Person or Family Members Have:

- Mental retardation or learning disabilities? If yes, is it progressive or non-progressive? (see Section 4.5)
- A large or small head?
- An unusually shaped head?
- Dysmorphic facial features? With particular focus on:
    Unusual placement/shape of eyes
    Synophrys (common in mucopolysaccharide storage disorders, de Lange syndrome)
    Unusual shape of nose
    Unusual shape/placement of ears
    Flat philtrum (common in fetal alcohol syndrome, de Lange syndrome)
    Coarsening of facial features (common in lysosomal storage disorders)
- Problems with hearing loss? (see Section 4.3)
- Problems with vision? (see Section 4.4)
    Congenital or juvenile cataracts (e.g., Cockayne syndrome, Smith–Lemli–Opitz syndrome) (see Tables 4.9 and 4.10)
    Blue sclerae (osteogenesis imperfecta, Hallerman–Streiff syndrome)
- Problems with the oral cavity (mouth/dentition)
    Cleft lip/palate
    Cleft palate (common in Kneist dysplasia, spondyloepiphyseal dysplasia congenita, diastrophic dysplasia)
    Unusual dentition

(continued)

TABLE 4.24   *(continued)*

- Hair anomalies?
    Hirsutism (common in de Lange syndrome, mucopolysaccharidoses, Rubinstein–Taybi
        syndrome)
    Sparse (seen in Dubowitz syndrome)
    Low posterior hairline (common in Turner and Noonan syndromes)
- A webbed neck? (common in Turner and Noonan syndromes)
- Hand/nail anomalies?
    Brachydactyly (common in several short stature syndromes including Aarskog
        syndrome)
    Postaxial polydactyly (common in chondroectodermal dysplasia, lethal short rib-
        polydactyly syndromes, asphyxiating thoracic dysplasia)
    Preaxial polydactyly (maternal diabetes, atelosteogenesis)
    Nail anomalies (hypoplastic in chondroectodermal dysplasia; hypoplastic or absent in
        sclerosteosis/Van Buchem disease, and Fanconi pancytopenia syndrome; short/broad
        in cartilage-hair hypoplasia/McKusick type of metaphyseal dysplasia)
    Broad thumbs (e.g., Rubinstein–Taybi syndrome)
- Feet anomalies?
    Clubfeet (e.g., spondyloepiphyseal dysplasia congenita, trisomy 18, diastrophic
        dysplasia)
- Skeletal involvement? (obtain all skeletal films!)
    Congenital dislocations or frequent postnatal dislocations
    Multiple fractures—Note age at onset and bones involved (e.g., osteogenesis
        imperfecta, congenital osteopetrosis, hypophosphatasia; osteopetrotic syndrome in
        older individuals with fractures)
    Scoliosis
    Pectus deformities
    Limb anomalies (common in many syndromes)
    Clubfeet (e.g., spondyloepiphyseal dysplasia congenita, trisomies 13 and 18)
    Arthrogryposis (congenital contractures) (seen in more than 120 syndromes, AD, AR, XL
        and chromosomal; and can also be attributed to maternal hyperthermia and
        infections)
- Unusual birth marks, rashes, or pigmentation? (common in Bloom syndrome, Fanconi
    pancytopenia syndrome)
- Congenital heart defects? (common in Turner syndrome, Noonan syndrome)
- Genital anomalies?
    Cryptorchidism (e.g., Smith–Lemli–Opitz syndrome)
    Hypospadias (e.g., Smith–Lemli–Opitz syndrome, Opitz syndrome, Dubowitz sydrome,
        de Lange syndrome, Fanconi pancytopenia syndrome)
    Small genitalia (e.g., Noonan syndrome, Robinow syndrome)
    "Shawl" scrotum (common in Aarskog syndrome)
- Infertility? (see Section 4.16)
- Seizures? (see section 4.8)
- Renal anomalies? (see section 4.13)
- Diabetes? (see Section 4.15)

Sources: Graham and Rimoin, 1997; Jones, 1997; Sanders, 1996.

chronic disease (particularly renal disease), a malabsorption disorder, endocrine/ metabolic disorders, a genetic or chromosomal syndrome, or a teratogenic exposure (Graham and Rimoin, 1997). If possible, obtain actual measurements of upper to lower body segment ratio, arm length, and sitting height rather than relying on a visual estimate; minor skeletal dysplasias such as hypochondroplasia are easy to miss (Graham and Rimoin, 1997).

The medical-family history questions to be asked when an individual has short stature are reviewed in Table 4.24. Medical-family history features of inherited metabolic disorders are reviewed in Table 4.11, and the features of chromosomal disorders in Table 3.2. In taking a family history, do not use the antiquated terms "dwarf" (in reference to an individual with disproportionate short stature) and "midget" (in reference to persons with proportionate short stature).

4.15 DIABETES

There are more than 70 syndromes associated with type I (insulin-dependent diabetes mellitus) and type II (noninsulin dependent diabetes mellitus). Type II diabetes is distinguished by diabetes of adult onset (usually after age 40 years), which is mostly managed with oral medication and/or diet, and is associated with obesity. Type I diabetes usually has onset of symptoms in childhood or as a young adult, and individuals require insulin for survival. Currently, genetic counseling is provided from empirical risk tables. In a given family, the type of diabetes "runs true," meaning that the immediate family members are at increased risk for the specific type of

TABLE 4.25 Medical-Family History Questions for Diabetes Mellitus

- What is the age of onset of diabetes? Are other family members affected?
- How is the diabetes managed? (e.g., With insulin injections? By diet, with or without oral medications?)
- Is the person overweight?
- Does the person use alcohol? How much and how often?
- Does the person have learning disabilities or mental retardation? If so, are they progressive or stable?
- Does this person have unusual facial features (dysmorphic)?
- Does the person or any family members have other diseases? Particularly:
  Visual disturbances? If yes, see Section 4.4.
  Hearing loss? If yes, see Section 4.3. The autosomal recessive Wolfram (DIDMOAD) syndrome is associated with juvenile onset diabetes, optic atrophy, and nerve deafness. It is thought to affect approximately 1 in 150 individuals with juvenile diabetes (Arnould and Hussels, 1997). Some of the mitochondrial myopathies are associated with diabetes mellitus and hearing loss (Wallace et al, 1997).
  Pancreatic disease? (common in cystic fibrosis and hemochromatosis)
  Pulmonary disease? (e.g., cystic fibrosis, alpha-1-antritypsin deficiency)
  Neurological problems? If yes, see Section 4.7.
  Neuromuscular disease? (several of the hereditary ataxias, muscular dystrophies, myotonic dystrophy, and mitochondrial myopathies are associated with diabetes mellitus)

Sources: Raffel et al., 1997; Rotter et al., 1992.

diabetes that has already occurred in a family member (Raffel et al., 1997). Raffel et al. (1997) and Rotter et al. (1992) provide good summaries of the many syndromes associated with diabetes mellitus. In most of these syndromes, diabetes is an important complication to be aware of for management purposes, but diabetes is seldom a presenting sign in the family history. Medical-family history questions for a family history of diabetes are given in Table 4.25.

4.16 REPRODUCTIVE FAILURE, INFERTILITY, AND MULTIPLE MISCARRIAGES

Approximately 10% of couples who wish to conceive experience infertility (Chandra and Stephen, 1998). Infertility is commonly defined as lack of conception after one year of unprotected intercourse. Infertility is a couple's disease; both partners must be throughly evaluated because male and female factors contribute almost equally (Greenhouse et al., 1998). Infertility may also reflect early spontaneous abortion rather than inability to conceive.

The risk of miscarriage for any recognized pregnancy is at least 15% (Garber et al., 1997). Any couple who has experienced three or more miscarriages should be evaluated for a chromosome anomaly. Any maternal condition that decreases uteroplacental blood flow may lead to fetal demise (e.g., hypertension, placental abruption from trauma, autoimmune disorders, diabetes mellitus). Miscarriages are also associated with a few maternal teratogenic agents (Garber et al., 1997) including:

- Coumarin derivatives
- Certain anticonvulsants
- Antineoplastic agents
- Alcohol and possibly tobacco use
- Cocaine use
- Retinoids
- Misoprostol

The most common causes of female infertility involve ovulatory dysfunction and fallopian tube disease. Mullerian duct anomalies are a rare cause of female infertility. Uterine fibroids may also play a role (Greenhouse et al., 1998). Structural chromosomal anomalies may be seen in women who have difficulty conceiving (Mau et al., 1997). There seem to be far fewer genetic causes of female infertility than male infertility (Chandley et al., 1997). Turner syndrome (45,X) is a rare but important cause of female infertility and is characterized (in adult women) by short stature, mild dysmorphic features, primary amennorhea, and failure of secondary sexual development. Women with triple X (47,XXX) may have menstrual irregularities, and can have problems with fertility. Women with primary ammenorhea may also have male pseudohermaphroditism (strictly defined as an individual with a Y chromosome whose external genitalia fail to develop as expected for a normal male) (Simpson, 1997). These individuals may be 45,X/46,XY mosaics. Individuals with X-linked testicular feminization (phenotypic females with a 46,XY karyotype) may also present with primary ammenorhea.

Infertility in men has been ascribed to multiple factors including (Chandley, 1997):

- Radiation or chemical exposure (such as from chemotherapy)
- Infection (such as infection of the accessory gland)
- Anatomic causes (e.g., obstructive disorders, varicocele)
- Endocrine causes
- Genetic disorders (see Table 4.26), including syndromes with hypogonadism as a feature
- Immunologic causes (antisperm antibodies)
- Idiopathic

TABLE 4.26 Genetic Causes of Male Infertility Where Infertility May be a Presenting Clinical Feature[a]

Condition	Inheritance Pattern[b]
Chromosomal	
Klinefelter syndrome (47,XXY)	Sporadic, chromosomal nondisjunction
Translocations of X or Y and an autosome	Sporadic or inherited
Autosomal translocations (Robertsonian and reciprocal)	Sporadic or inherited (test parents)
Chromosome inversions (pericentric)	Sporadic or inherited
Marker chromosomes	Sporadic
Microscopic Y-deletions	Yq11
Single gene	
Androgen insensitivity syndromes	XL
Congenital absence of vas deferens (CAVD)— cystic fibrosis (CFTR) mutations	AR
Globozoospermia (round-headed spermatozoa)	Unknown (rare)
Hemochromatosis	AR
Kallmann syndrome	AR, XL
Kartagener syndrome (immotile cilia syndrome)	AR
Myotonic dystrophy	AD
Noonan syndrome (if cryptorchidism)	AD
Sickle cell disease (hypothalamic-pituitary dysfunction)	AR
Spinobulbular muscular atrophy (Kennedy disease)	XL
Steroid sulfatase deficiency (X-linked ichthyosis)	XL
Young syndrome	AR

[a]Disorders where infertility is a feature but not usually a presenting sign are excluded.
[b]AD = autosomal dominant; AR = autosomal recessive; XL = X-linked.
Sources: Bonaccorsi et al., 1997; Chandley, 1997; Wieacker and Jakubiczka, 1997.

The first step in evaluating a man for infertility is semen analysis. Abnormalities in sperm motility, morphology, and concentration are particularly useful in assessing a genetic etiology for male infertility.

Approximately 11% of men with infertility have azoospermia or oligospermia. Within this group of men, there are several genetic factors to consider:

1. *Chromosome anomalies* (aneuploidy, sex chromosome mocaicism, and structural anomalies). Estimates are that between 4 and 7% of men with oligo-zoospermia or azoospermia have a structural chromosome anomaly (ring chromosome, reciprocal translocation, insertion, or inversion) (Bonaccorsi et al., 1997; Chandley, 1997; Johnson, 1998; Mau et al., 1997; McLaren, 1998). Klinefelter syndrome (47,XXY) is the most frequently observed chromosome anomaly in infertile men, affecting over 10% of men with azoospermia (Johnson, 1998).

2. *Cystic fibrosis* transmembrane conductance (CFTR) mutations in men with congenital absence of the vas deferens (CAVD). Approximately 1–2% of men with azoospermia have CAVD. Many (perhaps as high as 75%) of these men have CFTR mutations or mutations in disease-associated CFTR variants (such as the 5T allele) (Dork et al., 1997).

3. *Microscopic Y-deletions.* Specific Y-deletions have been identified in 10–15% of infertile men, and a genetic basis of infertility may exist (including autosomal loci) in many infertile men currently classified as having idiopathic infertility (Bhasin et al., 1997). Two Y-specific genes have been identified in infertile men—the AZF (azoospermia factor) gene and the DAZ (deleted-in-azoospermia) gene. Because these Y-microdeletions are also found in men with oligozoospermia, AZF and DAZ are misnomers (Kremer et al., 1997).

4. There may be *anomalies in the androgen receptor gene* on the X chromosome.

5. *Mitochondrial mutations* may be associated with asthenozoospermia (reduced sperm motility) (St John et al., 1997).

Suggestions for medical-family history questions for male infertility are given in Table 4.27.

Infertile men with normal semen parameters may also have genetic mechanisms for infertility. Some etiologies proposed from mouse models suggest there may be hereditary factors involved with the the ability of sperm to bind with the zona pellucida or with the later steps of sperm maturation (Okabe et al., 1998).

The potential heritability of infertility is an important topic to discuss with men with male-factor infertility undergoing ICSI (intracytoplasmic sperm injection) in order to conceive a pregnancy (Johnson, 1998; Kremer et al., 1997). From my observations, couples with male-factor infertility whom I have counseled prior to ICSI are much more concerned about passing on infertility to a future child than about possibly having a child with cystic fibrosis, even though a child with CF might be perceived as having more health burdens. Such couples undergo considerable emo-

TABLE 4.27 Medical-Family History Questions Related to Male Infertility

- What is the sperm count and sperm morphology? (obtain records)
- What is the man's height? (unusually tall stature suggestive of Klinefelter syndrome)
- Does the man have:
  Anything unusual about the way he looks? (wide-spaced eyes and other dysmorphic features characteristic of Noonan syndrome)
  A small penis?
  Small testes? (seen in many infertile males)
  Learning disabilities? (suggestive of Noonan, Kallman, and Klinefelter syndromes, and myotonic dystrophy)
  Any problems with his ability to smell? (seen in Klinefelter and Kallman syndromes)
  Nasal polyps? (seen in cystic fibrosis, Kartagener and Young syndromes)
  Chronic infections, asthma, pulmonary disease, sinus infections? (seen in cystic fibrosis, Kartagener and Young syndromes, chronic infections in cystic fibrosis and sickle cell disease)
  Any problems with muscle weakness? (myotonic dystrophy, spinal bulbar muscular atrophy, possible mitochondrial disease)
  Early cataracts? (myotonic dystrophy)
  Any unusual birthmarks, rashes, or scaling skin? (seen in X-linked icthyosis)
  "Bronze" skin coloration? (possible hemochromatosis)
  Any chronic diseases?
- Is there a family history of:
  Miscarriages? (possible parental chromosomal rearrangement)
  Learning disabilities or mental retardation? (possible chromosomal disorder, myotonic dystrophy, Noonan syndrome, Kallman syndrome)
  Anyone with multiple birth defects? (possible chromosomal disorder)
  Chronic infections, asthma, pulmonary disease, sinus infections? (cystic fibrosis, Kartagener and Young syndromes; chronic infections in sickle cell disease)
  Muscle disease? (myotonic dystrophy, spinal bulbar muscular atrophy)
- What is the man's ethnic background? (particularly useful to know for testing for cystic fibrosis mutations and screening for sickle cell anemia)
- Are the parents of the man related as cousins or more closely related?

tional and financial expense to arrive at a decision to undergo ICSI; they often think twice about the potential to place their future offspring at risk to suffer similar emotional heartache and frustrations in their future. The reproductive impact on the children conceived by ICSI will not be known for another 20–40 years when these individuals attempt to have their own families.

4.17 SUDDEN INFANT DEATH SYNDROME

Rarely, sudden infant death syndrome is the result of an inborn error of metabolism. Strictly defined, SIDS is the unexpected death of a "well" child over 1 month of age for which no explanation can be found despite postmortem examination. More than 30 autosomal recessive metabolic defects are candidate causes of SIDS (Saudubray and Charpentier, 1995). To rule out an inborn error of metabolism it is useful to obtain autopsy reports on the child, particularly looking for fatty changes in the liver, and skeletal and heart muscle. A history of illness before death (such as diarrhea, vomiting, and failure to thrive) might suggest a metabolic etiology. Consanguinity in the parents might also increase your suspicion of an inherited metabolic etiology because of an increased likelihood of autosomal recessive inheritance. Refer to Table 4.11 for the medical-family history features suggestive of an inborn error of metabolism.

REFERENCES

Aldred MA, Jay M, Wright AF (1994). X-linked retinitis pigmentosa. In Wright AF, Jay B (eds), *Molecular Genetics of Inherited Eye Disorders*. Switzerland: Harwood Academic Publishers, p. 259.

American Association on Mental Retardation (1992). *Mental Retardation—Definition, Classification, and Systems of Supports Workbook*. Washington, DC: American Association on Mental Retardation.

American College of Medical Genetics (ACMG) (1998). Statement on folic acid: fortification and supplementation. Genetics In Med 1:66.

American College of Medical Genetics/American Society of Human Genetics (ACMG/ASHG) Huntington Disease Genetic Testing Working Group (1998). Laboratory guidelines for Huntington disease genetic testing. Am J Hum Genet 62:1243–1247.

Arnould VJ, Hussels IE (1997). Optic atrophy and congenital blindness. In Rimoin DL, Connor JM, Pyeritz RE (eds), *Emery & Rimoin's Principles and Practice of Medical Genetics*, 3rd ed. New York: Churchill Livingstone, pp. 2487–2503.

Baraitser M (1997). *The Genetics of Neurological Disorders*. Oxford: Oxford University Press.

Berry GT, Bennett MJ (1998). A focused approach to diagnosing inborn errors of metabolism. Contem Ped 15:79–102.

Bérubé M (1996). *Life As We Know It: A Father, a Family and an Exceptional Child*. New York: Pantheon Books.

Bhasin S, Ma K, de Kretser DM (1997). Y-chromosome microdeletions and male infertility. Ann Med 29:261–263.

Bird TD (1992). Epilepsy. In King RA, Rotter JI, Motulsky AG (eds), *The Genetic Basis of Common Diseases*. New York: Oxford University Press, pp. 732–752.

Bonaccorsi AC, Martins RRS, Vargas FR, Franco JG, Botler J (1997). Genetic disorders in normally androgenized infertile men and the use of intracytoplasmic sperm injection as a way of treatment. Fertil Steril 67:928–931.

Bryson SE (1996). Brief report: epidemiology of autism. J Autism Dev Disorder 26:165–167.

Bundey S (1997). Abnormal mental development. In Rimoin DL, Connor JM, Pyeritz RE (eds), *Emery and Rimoin's Principles and Practice of Medical Genetics*, 3rd ed. New York: Churchill Livingstone, pp. 725–736.

Burn J, Goodship J (1997). Congenital heart disease. In Rimoin DL, Connor JM, Pyeritz RE (eds), *Emery and Rimoin's Principles and Practice of Medical Genetics*, 3rd ed. New York: Churchill Livingstone, pp. 767–828.

Carlson C, Papolos D, Pandita RK, et al. (1997). Molecular analysis of velo-cardio-facial syndrome patients with psychiatric disorders. Am J Hum Genet 60:851–859.

Chandley AC (1997). Infertility. In Rimoin DL, Connor JM, Pyeritz RE (eds), *Emery and Ri-*

moin's Principles and Practice of Medical Genetics, 3rd ed. New York: Churchill Livingstone, pp. 667–675.

Chandra A, Stephen EH (1998). Impaired fecundity in the United States: 1982—1996. Fam Plann Perspect 30:34–42.

Clarke JTR (1996). *A Clinical Guide to Inherited Metabolic Diseases*. Great Britain: Cambridge University Press.

Cohen MM, Gorlin RJ (1995). Epidemiology, etiology, and genetic patterns. In Gorlin RJ, Toriello HV, Cohen MM (eds), *Hereditary Hearing Loss and Its Syndromes*. New York, Oxford: Oxford University Press, pp. 9–21.

Cohen MM (1997). *The Child with Multiple Birth Defects*. Oxford: Oxford University Press.

Cohen MM, Gorlin RJ, Fraser FC (1997). Craniofacial disorders. In Rimoin DL, Connor JM, Pyeritz RE (eds), *Emery and Rimoin's Principles and Practice of Medical Genetics*, 3rd ed. New York: Churchill Livingstone, pp. 1121–1147.

Cook EH, Courchesne RY, Cox NJ, et al. (1998). Linkage-disequilibrium mapping of autistic disorder, with 5q11–13 markers. Am J Hum Genet 62:1077–1083.

Coonar AS, McKenna WJ (1997). Molecular genetics of familial cardiomyopathies. Advan Genet 35:285–324.

Cremers FPM (1998). Genetic causes of hearing loss. Curr Opin Neurol 11:11–16.

Czeizel AE, T'oth M, Rockenbauer M (1996). Population-based case control study of folic acid supplementation during pregnancy. Teratology 53:345–351.

Dork T, Dworniczak B, Aulehla-Scholz C, et al. (1997). Distinct spectrum of CFTR gene mutations in congenital absence of vas deferens. Hum Genet 100:365–377.

Elmslie F, Gardiner M (1997). The epilepsies. In Rimoin DL, Connor JM, Pyeritz RE (eds), *Emery and Rimoin's Principles and Practice of Medical Genetics*, 3rd ed. New York: Churchill Livingstone, pp. 2177–2196.

Emery AEH (1998). *Neuromuscular Disorders: Clinical and Medical Genetics*. New York: Wiley-Liss.

Eydoux P, Khalife S (1997). Prenatal diagnosis. In Tewfik TL, Der Kaloustian VM (eds), *Congenital Anomalies of the Ear, Nose, and Throat*. New York: Oxford University Press, pp. 67–75.

Finucane B (1998). *Working with Women Who Have Mental Retardation: A Genetic Counselor's Guide*. Pennsylvania: Elwyn, Inc.

Fischel-Ghodsian N, Falk RE (1997). Deafness. In Rimoin DL, Connor JM, Pyeritz RE (eds), *Emery & Rimoin's Principles and Practice of Medical Genetics*, 3rd ed. New York: Churchill Livingstone, pp. 1149–1170.

Garber AP, Schreck R, Carlson DE (1997). Fetal loss. In Rimoin DL, Connor JM, Pyeritz RE (eds), *Emery & Rimoin's Principles and Practice of Medical Genetics*, 3rd ed. New York: Churchill Livingstone, pp. 677–686.

Gorlin RJ, Cohen M, Levin LS (1990). *Syndromes of the Head and Neck,* 3rd ed. New York: Oxford University Press.

Gorlin RJ, Toriello HV, Cohen MM (1995). *Hereditary Hearing Loss and Its Syndromes*. New York: Oxford University Press.

Graham JM, Rimoin DL (1997). Abnormal body size and proportion. In Rimoin DL, Connor JM, Pyeritz RE (eds), *Emery and Rimoin's Principles and Practice of Medical Genetics*, 3rd ed. New York: Churchill Livingstone, pp. 737–752.

Greenhouse S, Ranking T, Dean J (1998). Insights from model systems. Genetic causes of female infertility: targeted mutagenesis in mice. Am J Hum Genet 62:1282–1287.

Hanson DR, Gottesman II (1992). Schizophrenia. In King RA, Rotter JI, Motulsky AG (eds), *The Genetic Basis of Common Diseases.* New York: Oxford University Press, pp. 816–836.

Heckenlively JR, Daiger SP (1997). Hereditary retinal and choroidal degenerations. In Rimoin DL, Connor JM, Pyeritz RE (eds), *Emery & Rimoin's Principles and Practice of Medical Genetics,* 3rd ed. New York: Churchill Livingstone, pp. 2555–2576.

Heston LI (1992). Alzheimer's disease. In King RA, Rotter JI, Motulsky AG (eds), *The Genetic Basis of Common Diseases.* New York: Oxford University Press, pp. 792–800.

Israel J, Cunningham M, Thumann H, Arnos KS (1996). Deaf Culture. In Fisher NL (ed), *Cultural and Ethnic Diversity: A Guide for Genetics Professionals.* Baltimore: Johns Hopkins University Press, pp. 220–239.

Johnson MD (1998). Genetic risk of intracytoplasmic sperm injection in the treatment of male infertility: recommendations for genetic counseling and screening. Fertil Steril 70:397–411.

Jones KL (1997). *Smith's Recognizable Patterns of Human Malformation,* 5th ed. Philadelphia: W. B. Saunders, Co.

Kalter H, Warkany J (1983). Congenital malformations—etiologic factors and their role in prevention. N Engl J Med. 308:424–431, 491–497 (2 parts).

Kelley PM, Harris DJ, Comer BC, et al. (1998). Novel mutations in the connexin 26 gene (GJB2) that cause autosomal recessive DFNB1 hearing loss. Am J Hum Genet 62:792–799.

Kendler KS (1997). The genetic epidemiology of psychiatric disorders: a current perspective. Soc Psychiatry Psychiatr Epidemiol 32:5–11.

Kendler KS, Silberg JL, Neale MC, Kessler RC, Heath AC, Eaves LJ (1991). The family history method: whose psychiatric history is measured? Am J Psychiatry 148:1501–1504.

Khoury MJ, Oliney RS, Rickson JD (1997). Epidemiology. In Tewfik TL, Der Kaloustian VM (eds), *Congenital Anomalies of the Ear, Nose, and Throat.* New York: Oxford University Press, pp. 47–56.

Kinney DK (1997). Schizophrenia. In Rimoin DL, Connor JM, Pyeritz RE (eds), *Emery & Rimoin's Principles and Practice of Medical Genetics,* 3rd ed. New York: Churchill Livingstone, pp. 1827–1841.

Kremer J, Tuerlings J, Meueleman E, et al. (1997). Microdeletions of the Y choromosome and intracytoplasmic sperm injection: from gene to clinic. Hum Repr 12(4):687–791.

Lashley FR (1998). *Clinical Genetics in Nursing Practice,* 2nd ed. New York: Springer Publishing Company.

Mau UA, Bäckert IT, Kaiser P, Kiesel L (1997). Chromosomal findings in 150 couples referred for genetic counselling prior to intracytoplasmic sperm injection. Hum Repro 12:930–937.

MacKinnon DF, Jamison KR, DePaulo JR (1997). Genetics of manic depressive illness. Annu Rev Neurosci 20:355–373.

McLaren A (1998). Genetics and human reproduction. Trends Genet 14:427–431.

Middleton A, Hewison J, Mueller RF (1998). Attitudes of deaf adults toward genetic testing for hereditary deafness. Am J Hum Genet 63:1175–1180.

Morgan S, Grunfeld J (eds) (1998). *Inherited Disorders of the Kidney.* New York: Oxford University Press.

Online Mendelian Inheritance in Man, OMIM (TM). Center for Medical Genetics, Johns Hopkins University (Baltimore, MD) and National Center for Biotechnology Information, National Library of Medicine (Bethesda, MD), 1997. Worldwide Web URL:http://www.ncbi.nlm.nih.gov/omim/

Okabe M, Ikawa M, Ashkenas J (1998). Gametogenesis '98. Male infertility and the genetics of spermatogenesis. Am J Hum Genet 62:1274–1281.

Pollen DA (1993). *Hannah's Heirs. The Quest for the Genetic Origins of Alzheimer's Disease.* New York: Oxford University Press.

Rabinowitz YS, Cotlier E, Park S (1997). Anomalies of the lens. In Rimoin DL, Connor JM, Pyeritz RE (eds), *Emery & Rimoin's Principles and Practice of Medical Genetics*, 3rd ed. New York: Churchill Livingstone, pp. 2535–2554.

Raffel LJ, Scheuner MT, Rimoin DL, Rotter JI (1997). Diabetes mellitus. In Rimoin DL, Connor JM, Pyeritz RE (eds), *Emery & Rimoin's Principles and Practice of Medical Genetics*, 3rd ed. New York: Churchill Livingstone, pp. 1401–1440.

Resta RG (1997). Carolyn's feet. Am J Med Genet 72:1–2.

Robinson A, Linden MG (1993). *Clinical Genetics Handbook,* 2nd ed. Boston: Blackwell Scientific Publications.

Rodier PM, Bryson SE, Welch JP (1997). Minor malformation and physical measurements in autism: data from Nova Scotia. Teratology 55:319–325.

Roses AD, Pericak-Vance (1997). Alzheimer disease and other dementias. In Rimoin DL, Connor JM, Pyeritz RE (eds), *Emery & Rimoin's Principles and Practice of Medical Genetics*, 3rd ed. New York: Churchill Livingstone, pp. 1807–1825.

Rotter JI, Vadheim CM, Rimoin DL (1992). Diabetes mellitus. In King RA, Rotter JI, Motulsky AG (eds), *The Genetic Basis of Common Diseases*. New York: Oxford University Press, pp. 413–481.

Rubinstein WS (1997). A 'normal' practice. JAMA 278(15):1216.

Rutter M, Bailey A, Bolton P, Le Couteur A (1994). Autism and known medical conditions: myth and substance. J Child Psychol Psychiatry 35:311–322.

Sanders RC (ed) (1996). *Structural Fetal Abnormalities: The Total Picture*. St Louis: Mosby Yearbook, Inc.

Saudubray JM, Charpentier C (1995). Clinical phenotypes: diagnosis/algorithms. In Scriver CR, Beaudet AL, Sly WS, Valle D (eds), *The Metabolic and Molecular Bases of Inherited Disease,* 7th ed. New York: McGraw-Hill, pp. 327–400.

Schievink WI (1998). Genetics and aneurysm formation. Neurosurg Clin N Am 9:485–495.

Schwartz CE, Dean J, Howard-Peebles PN, et al. (1994). Obstetrical and gynecological complications in fragile X carriers: a multicenter study. Am J Med Genet 51:400–402.

Scriver CR, Beaudet AL, Sly WS, Valle D (eds) (1995). *The Metabolic and Molecular Bases of Inherited Disease*, 7th ed. New York: McGraw-Hill.

Seashore MR, Wappner RS (1996). *Genetics in Primary Care and Clinical Medicine.* Stamford: Appelton & Lange.

Shaw GM, Wasserman CR, Lammer EJ, et al. (1996). Orofacial clefts, parental cigarette smoking, and transforming growth factor-alpha gene variants. Am J Hum Genet 58:551–561.

Shprintzen RJ, Wang F, Goldberg R, Marion R (1985). The expanded velo-cardio-facial syndrome (VCF): additional features of the most common clefting syndrome. Am J Hum Genet 37:A77.

Simonoff E, Rutter M (1997). Autism and other behavioral disorders. In Rimoin DL, Connor JM, Pyeritz RE (eds), *Emery & Rimoin's Principles and Practice of Medical Genetics*, 3rd ed. New York: Churchill Livingstone, pp. 1791–

Simpson JL (1997). Disorders of the gonads, genital tract, and genitalia. In Rimoin DL, Connor JM, Pyeritz RE (eds), *Emery & Rimoin's Principles and Practice of Medical Genetics*, 3rd ed. New York: Churchill Livingstone, pp. 1477–1500.

Snijders RJM, Nicholaides KH (1997). Ultrasound markers for fetal chromosome defects. New York: Parthenon Publishing Group.

St John JC, Cook ID, Barratt CL (1997). Mitochondrial mutations and male infertility. Nat Med 3:124–125.

Sutherland GR, Mulley JC (1997). Fragile X syndrome and other causes of X-linked mental handicap. In Rimoin DL, Connor JM, Pyeritz RE (eds), *Emery & Rimoin's Principles and Practice of Medical Genetics*, 3rd ed. New York: Churchill Livingstone, pp. 1745–1766.

Sybert VP (1997). *Genetic Skin Disorders*. New York: Oxford University Press.

Taybi H, Lachman RS (1996). *Radiology of Syndromes, Metabolic Disorders, and Skeletal Dysplasias*, 4th ed. St. Louis: Mosby.

Tewfik TL, Teebi AS, Der Kaloustian VM (1997). Syndromes and conditions associated with genetic deafness. In Tewfik TL, Der Kaloustian VM (eds). *Congenital Anomalies of the Ear, Nose, and Throat*. New York: Oxford University Press.

Tolarova M, Harris J (1995). Reduced recurrence of orofacial clefts after periconceptional supplementation with high-dose folic acid and multivitamins. Teratology 51:71–78.

Tolmie J (1997). Neural tube defects and other congenital malformations of the central nervous system. In Rimoin DL, Connor JM, Pyeritz RE (eds), *Principles and Practice of Medical Genetics*, 3rd ed. New York: Churchill Livingstone, pp. 2145–2176.

Van Allen MI (1997). Congenital disorders of the urinary tract. In: *Emery & Rimoin's Principles and Practice of Medical Genetics*, 3rd ed. New York: Churchill Livingstone, pp. 2611–2641.

Van Camp G, Smith RJH. Hereditary Hearing Loss Homepage. World Wide Web, last updated 5-Nov-1998, URL: http://dnalab-www.uia.ac.be/dnalab/hhh/

Wallace DC, Brown MD, Lott MT (1997). Mitochondrial genetics. In Rimoin DL, Connor JM, Pyeritz RE (eds), *Principles and Practice of Medical Genetics*, 3rd ed. New York: Churchill Livingstone, pp. 277–332.

Wieacker P, Jakubiczka S (1997). Genetic causes of male infertility. Andrologia 29:63–69.

Wing L (1993). The definition and prevalence of autism. A review. Eur Child Adolesc Psychiatry 2:61–74.

Winter RM, Knowles SAS, Bieber FR, Baraitser M (1988). *The Malformed Fetus and Stillbirth*. New York: John Wiley & Sons.

5

Using a Pedigree to Recognize Individuals with an Increased Susceptibility to Cancer

> *I just returned home from the hospital, having had a small cyst removed from my right breast. Second time. It was benign. . . . My scars portend my lineage. I look at Mother and I see myself. Is cancer my path, too? . . . I belong to a Clan of One-Breasted Women. My mother, my grandmothers, and six aunts have all had mastectomies. Seven are dead. . . . This is my family history.*
> —*Terry Tempest Williams (1991)*

Every cancer is due to genetic mechanisms that have gone awry in the normal life cycle of cells, but most cancer is not inherited. Of all cancers, about 5–10% are thought to be due to hereditary syndromes. In comparison, approximately 30% of all cancers are associated with tobacco exposure (Offit, 1998). It is likely that an array of modifying genes and environmental factors influence each individual's risk of developing cancer.

A pedigree is the most cost-effective tool for identifying individuals who may have a higher susceptibility to cancer than their age-related background risk because of genetic factors. Inherited cancer syndromes have several key medical-family history features as shown in Table 5.1. Because taking a pedigree is time consuming, a brief cancer family history screening form (such as the one in Appendix A.3) is helpful for screening seemingly low-risk individuals. A more extensive history in the form of a pedigree can then be obtained on individuals with positive responses on the screening questionnaires that raise suspicion of a familial cancer syndrome. Table 5.2 reviews the screening questions for individuals with a family history of cancer.

TABLE 5.1   Medical-Family History Features Suggestive of a Hereditary Cancer Syndrome or a Site-specific Inherited Cancer Susceptibility

Multiple closely related individuals with cancer (of any type)
Pattern of affected individuals in family follows autosomal dominant model
Early age of onset of cancer (i.e., premenopausal breast cancer, colon cancer age <45–50 years, prostate cancer age <50–60 years, or childhood tumors)
Bilateral disease in paired organs
More than one primary tumor
Rare cancers (i.e., lung cancer in a nonsmoker, male breast cancer, or adrenocortical carcinoma)
Clusters of rare cancers in multiple individuals in a family (e.g., thyroid cancer)
Absence of occupational or environmental risk factors

TABLE 5.2   Medical-Family History Queries for Cancer[a]

Questions Related to Cancer

- Type of cancer(s) (document with pathology reports)
- Age at diagnosis of cancer
  Age of menopause (in individuals with breast cancer)
- If more than one cancer, was it a metastasis or a new primary? (obtain pathology reports)
- Bilateral cancers
- Treatment or management (i.e., chemotherapy, radiation, mastectomy, oophorectomy, colectomy)
- Presence of colonic polyps (get an estimate of how many polyps and obtain any pathology reports)
- Childhood cancers (LFS, FAP, JP, WTS, RB)
- Potential occupational exposures (see Table 5.7)
- Potential environmental exposures including alcohol and tobacco use (see Table 5.7)

General Family History Questions

- Ages of all *living* family members
- Age at death, and cause of death, for *all* family members
- Biopsies in any family member (confirm with pathology reports)
- Surgical procedures (including prophylactic) in *any* family member (e.g., mastectomy, oophorectomy, hysterectomy, colectomy)
- Chronic diseases in the family (particularly gastrointestinal disorders such as Crohn disease, ulcerative colitis)
- Ethnicity (ask specifically if Ashkenazi Jewish)

Targeted Medical Systems Review

- Blindness or eye tumors (RB, WTS, VHL, TS)
- Skin changes, birthmarks
  Café au lait in NF1
  Shagreen patches and ash leaf hypopigmented macules in TS
  Brown/black macules in PJS (perioral, buccal mucosa, palms, and fingers)
  Facial tricholemmomas (tan-yellow verrucous papules) in CS
  Multiple moles (dysplastic nevi) in melanoma susceptibility syndromes
  Bronzing or graying of skin (history of hepatocellular carcinoma secondary to hemochromatosis)
  Unusual pigmentation around the mouth (PJS, CS)

(continued)

TABLE 5.2 *(continued)*

- "Lumps and bumps"
  Fibromas in NF, CS, and FAP
  Periungual fibromas in TS
  Lipomas in CS, FAP, and MEN1
  Epidermoid cysts in FAP
  Adenoma sebaceum/angiofibromas in TS and MEN1
  Basal cell carcinomas- multiple dome-shaped skin-colored to tan papules in NBCCS
  Punctate keratoses on palms and soles in CS
- Lips "full" or "blubbery" (MEN2)
- Unusual "lumps" on tongue (mucosal neuromas in MEN2; papillomas in CS)
- Pitting in palms of the hands (CS, NBCCS)
- Hearing loss (NF2, VHL)
- Jaw cysts (osteomas) (FAP, NBCCS)
- Macrocephaly (large head) (NBCCS, sometimes in NF1, CS)
- Leukemia (LFS)
- Thyroid disease/cancer (FMTC, MEN2, CS)
- Uterine fibroids (CS)
- Ovarian cysts (CS, PJS)
- Mental retardation/learning disabilities with or without dysmorphic features (CS, WTS, TS, NF1, NBCCS)
- Peptic ulcers (MEN1)
- Diabetes (associated with pancreatic cancer)
- Seizures (possible CNS tumor)
- Male breast cancer—ask about fertility (possibility of Klinefelter–XXY syndrome)

*a*Abbreviations: BOC = Breast-ovarian cancer; CS = Cowden syndrome; FAP = familial adenomatous polyposis; LFS = Li–Fraumeni syndrome; MEN = multiple endocrine neoplasia; NF = neurofibromatosis; NBCCS = nevoid basal cell carcinoma syndrome (Gorlin syndrome); PJS = Peutz–Jeghers syndromes; RB = retinoblastoma, TS = tuberous sclerosis; VHL = von Hippel–Lindau syndrome; WTS = Wilms' tumor syndromes

Options for genetic testing and increased cancer surveillance are based on the patient's placement in the pedigree in relation to relatives affected with cancer. Information gleaned from a patient's physical examination and pedigree analysis (with or without molecular testing) provides the clinician with fodder for discourse with the patient about multiple health issues. Recommendations can be made regarding age of initiation (and method) of cancer screening; encouraging healthy life-style choices (i.e., diet, exercise, use of alcohol and tobacco products, hormone therapies); possibly even occupational choices and surgical interventions (Burke, Daly et al., 1997; Burke, Petersen et al., 1997; Offit, 1998). Individuals who may benefit from cancer genetic counseling include healthy persons with a family history of cancer and those with cancer who are concerned about their risks of having another primary malignancy or the chances their offspring may develop cancer.

The focus of this chapter is to identify the signposts in the medical-family history that are clues to identifying the growing number of autosomal dominant familial cancer susceptibility syndromes (refer to Table 5.3). Many of these cancer susceptibility syndromes include more than one common site of malignancy (for example, hereditary non-polyposis coli is primarily associated with cancers of the colon,

TABLE 5.3   Known Autosomal Dominant Cancer Predisposition Syndromes and Their Gene Locations

Autosomal Dominant Cancer Predisposition Syndromes	Gene Locus (loci)
Acute myelocytic leukemia	16q, 21q
Cowden syndrome (CS)	PTEN (10q22-23)
Familial adenomatous polyposis coli (FAP)	APC (5q21-q22)
Familial atypical multiple-mole melanoma (FAMMM)	p16 (CDKN2)
Familial juvenile polyposis (FJP or JPC)	18q21.1?
Familial medullary thyroid carcinoma (FMTC)	RET (10q11.2)
Familial prostate cancer (FPC)	probably multiple loci
Gastric polyposis	unknown
Hereditary clear-cell renal carcinoma (HCRC)	unknown
Hereditary melanoma (HM)	1p36, CDKN (9p21), CDK4 (6q)
Hereditary mixed-polyposis syndrome	6q?
Hereditary non-polyposis colon cancer (HNPCC)	MSH2 (2p15) and MLH1 (3p21) are most common, others: MSH6 (2p16), PMS1 (2q31), PMS2 (7p22)
Hereditary papillary renal carcinoma (HPRC)	MET (7q31.1-34)
Hereditary breast-ovarian cancer syndrome (HBOC)	BRCA1 (17q21), BRCA2 (13q12-13)
Li–Fraumeni syndrome (LFS)	p53 (17p.13.1)
Muir–Torre syndrome	MSH2, MLH1
Multiple endocrine neoplasia 1 (MEN1)	MEN1 11q13
Multiple endocrine neoplasia 2 (MEN2A, 2B)	RET (10q11.2)
Neuroblastoma	NB
Neurofibromatosis 1 (NF1)	NF1 (17q11.2)
Neurofibromatosis 2 (NF2)	NF2 (22q12.2)
Nevoid basal cell carcinoma syndrome (NBCCS)	PTCH 9q31
Papillary thyroid carcinoma	unknown
Peutz–Jeghers syndrome (PJS)	STK11/LKB1 (19p13.3), 19q13.4?
Retinoblastoma	RB1 (13q14)
Tuberous sclerosis (types 1 and 2) (TS)	type 1 (9q32-q34), type 2 (16p13.3)
Turcot–FAP variant	APC (5q21-q22)
Turcot–HNPCC variant	MLH1, MSH2
Von Hippel–Lindau (VHL) syndrome	VHL 3p25-p26
Wilms' tumor	WT-1

Sources: Akiyama et al., 1997; Cummings and Olufunmilayo, 1998; Eng and Ji, 1998; Flanders and Foulkes, 1996; Foulkes and Hodgson, 1998; Hemminki et al., 1998; Hisada M et al., 1998; Howe et al., 1998; Jacoby et al., 1997; Jenne et al., 1998; Liaw et al., 1997; Lynch ED et al., 1997; Lynch HT et al., 1997; Mehenni et al., 1997; Miyaki et al., 1997; Offit, 1998; Olschwang et al., 1998; Schmidt et al., 1997; Vogelstein and Kinzler, 1998

stomach, uterus, and ovary). Some cancer susceptibility syndromes involve other medical features besides neoplasm. Cowden syndrome is associated with breast and thyroid carcinoma, thyroid disease, benign hamartomas, and specific dermatologic findings. Tables 5.4a and 5.4b correlate the neoplasms, benign tumors, and other physical features that are associated with many of the autosomal dominant cancer susceptibility syndromes listed in Table 5.3. Tables 5.4a and 5.4b are resources for

TABLE 5.4a   Autosomal Dominant Cancer Syndromes and their Associations with Benign Tumors and Neoplasms

Benign Tumors and Malignancies	Syndromes[a]						
	LFS	HBOC1	HBOC2	PJS	CS	HNPCC	FAP
Ocular							
CHRPE							X
Ocular melanoma			?				
Brain/CNS tumors							
Brain tumors—all types	X						
Astrocytoma	X						
Cerebellar gangliocytomas					?		
Glioblastoma	X					X[b]	
Glioma	X				X		
Meningioma					X		
Medulloblastoma	X						X[b]
Neuroblastoma	?						
Endocrine							
Adrenocortical tumors	X						
Thyroid adenomas					X		
Follicular thyroid adenocarcinoma					X		
Thyroid carcinoma—papillary					?	?	
Respiratory							
Nasal polyps				X			
Laryngeal carcinoma	?		?				
Lung adenocarcinoma	?				?		
Reproductive							
Breast fibroadenomas					X	?	
Breast cancer	X	X	X[c]	X	X	?	
Ovarian cancer	?	X	X	?	?	X	
Uterine cancer				?	?	X	
Uterine leiomyoma					X		
Cervical cancer	?			?	?	?	
Testicular cancer	?			?		?	
Gastrointestinal							
Gastric cancer				X	?	X	X
Gastrointestinal cancer				X	?	X	X
Colorectal cancer—polyposis							X
Colorectal cancer—non-polyposis	?	?	?	X		X[d]	
Colonic hamartomas					X	X	
Prostate cancer	?	X	X				
Genitourinary							
Transitional cell tumors of renal pelvis or ureter						X	
Pancreatic cancer	?	?	?	X[b]	?	X[b]	?
Connective tissue							
Osteosarcoma	X						
Soft-tissue sarcomas	X						
Rhabdomyosarcomas	X						
Hematologic and lymphatic							
Hematologic malignancy	X	?					
Skin							
Melanoma	?	?			?		

(continued)

TABLE 5.4a *(continued)*

	Syndromes[a]						
Benign Tumors and Malignancies	LFS	HBOC1	HBOC2	PJS	CS	HNPCC	FAP
Other							
Cutaneous findings				X	X	X[b]	X
Learning disabilities/MR					X[b]		
Macrocephaly					X[b]		

Abbreviations: LFS = Li–Fraumeni syndrome; HBOC1 = hereditary breast ovarian cancer syndrome 1; HBOC2 = hereditary breast ovarian cancer syndrome 2; PJS = Peutz–Jeghers syndrome; CS = Cowden syndrome; HNPCC = hereditary non-polyposis coli syndrome; FAP = familial adenomatous polyposis coli; CHRPE = congenital hypertrophy of the retinal pigment epithelium; ? = associations that are not well characterized or are controversial.
[b]Recognized but uncommon manifestation.
[c]Includes male breast cancer.
[d]Predominantly right-sided (proximal) colonic cancer.
Source: Refer to Table 5.3 for the sources for this table.

helping to recognize a potential hereditary cancer syndrome when a cluster of cancers is found in a family history.

Increased risk for malignancy is a secondary characteristic of more than 100 single gene and chromosomal disorders (Friedman, 1997; Schneider, 1994). For most of these conditions, knowledge about increased risk for neoplasm is important for the lifelong health management of these individuals, but cancer is unlikely to be the presenting diagnostic feature (i.e., leukemia in Down syndrome or adenocarcinoma of the ileum in cystic fibrosis). Listed in Table 5.5 are examples of some of the more well-known genetic syndromes associated with neoplasms and their modes of inheritance. With the exception of hemochromatosis, most of the syndromes in Table 5.5 are diagnosed in childhood.

Our knowledge about the phenotypes of the familial cancer syndromes is in continual flux as the tools of molecular genetics continue to define the germ line mutations associated with particular cancer syndromes. For example, Turcot syndrome (a rare condition with brain tumors and colon cancers) is now known to be associated with germline mutations in at least three separate genes—the adenomatous polyposis coli (APC) gene (at 5q21-q22); and two of the hereditary non-polyposis coli (HNPCC)-associated mutations, MLH1 (at 3p21) and PMS2 (at 7p22). Mutations in the APC gene are associated with medulloblastoma, and HNPCC mutations are correlated with glioblastoma (Offit, 1998). Until recently, mutations in the PTEN gene (at 10q22-q23) were thought to be responsible for three rare disorders (juvenile polyposis syndrome, Cowden syndrome, and Bannayan–Zonana or Bannayan–Riley–Ruvalcaba syndrome) that have intestinal hamartomas, lipomas, macrocephaly, and other features (Jacoby et al., 1997, Liaw et al., 1997; Lynch, Ostermeyer et al., 1997; Marsh et al., 1997; Offit, 1998; Olschwang et al., 1998). Upon further molecular analysis, it is now believed that juvenile polyposis syndrome is a separate entity, with mutations in 18q21.1 and possibly other loci (Howe et al., 1998). Those individuals with a PTEN mutation who seem to have the pheno-

TABLE 5.4b Autosomal Dominant Cancer Syndromes (continued)

Benign Tumors/Growths and Malignancies	MEN1	MEN2	NF1	NF2	NBCCS	TS	VHL	FAMMM
Ocular								
Retinal angioma							X	
Retinal hamartomas				X		X		
Iris hamartomas (Lish nodules)			X					
Optic glioma			X					
Oral/gastrointesinal								
Jaw cysts					X			
Mucosal neuromas		X						
Gastrointestinal malignancies								X
Brain/CNS Tumors								
Endolymphatic sac tumor							X	
Vestibular schwannomas—bilateral				X				
Astrocytoma			X[b]	X		X		
Ependymoma				X[b]		X[b]		
Glioma				X				
Hemangioblastoma							X	
Meningioma				X	X[b]			
Medulloblastoma					X[b]			
Endocrine								
Parathyroid adenoma	X		X					
Pituitary adenoma	X							
Thyroid carcinoma—medullary		X						
Respiratory								
Lung adenocarcinoma							?	X
Cardiovascular								
Cardiac rhabdomyoma						X		
Reproductive								
Ovarian fibrosarcoma					X[b]			
Epididymal cystadenoma							X	
Genitourinary								
Renal cell carcinoma—clear cell						X	X	
Angiomyolipoma						X		
Pheochromocytoma		X	X[b]				X	
Pancreatic islet cell tumors	X						X[b]	
Pancreatic cancer							X[b]	X[b]
Connective tissue								
Rhabdomyosarcoma			X[b]					
Neurofibrosarcoma			X[b]	?				
Skin								
Basal cell carcinoma					X			
Melanoma								X
Neurofibroma			X	X[b]				
Multiple nevi								X
Other								
Cutaneous findings			X	X[b]	X	X		X
Learning disabilities/MR			X[b]		X[b]	X		
Macrocephaly			X[b]		X			

[a]Abbreviations: MEN1 = multiple endocrine neoplasia 1; MEN2 = multiple endocrine neoplasia 2; NF1 = neurofibromatosis 1; NF2 = neurofibromatosis 2; NBCCS = nevoid basal cell carcinoma syndrome; TS = tuberous sclerosis complex; VHL = von Hippel–Lindau syndrome; FAMMM = familial atypical multiple-mole melanoma; ? = associations that are not well characterized or are controversial.

[b]Recognized but uncommon manifestation.

Source: Refer to Table 5.3 for the sources for this table.

TABLE 5.5 Selected Genetic Syndromes Associated with Neoplasms and Their Inheritance Patterns

Inheritance Pattern	Neoplasm	Syndrome[a]
Autosomal Dominant	Wilms' tumor	Hereditary Wilms' tumor syndromes
	Retinoblastoma	Hereditary retinoblastoma
	Chondrosarcoma	Hereditary multiple exostoses syndromes
	Hepatocellular carcinoma	Alpha-1-antitrypsin deficiency (chronic lung disease, juvenile cirrhosis and liver disease)
Autosomal recessive	Multiple neoplasms	Bloom syndrome (growth deficiency, DD, erythema with telangiectasias on face and neck, characteristic facies, hypogonadism)
	Leukemia and lymphoma	Ataxia telangiectasia (progressive ataxia with choreoathetosis, multiple telangiectasia, immunodeficiency, DD)
	Leukemia and hepatocellular carcinoma	Fanconi syndrome (pancytopenia, radial ray defects with multiple congenital anomalies, DD, deafness)
	Multiple cutaneous malignancies	Xeroderma pigmentosum (acute hypersensitivity to sun with invariable cutaneous malignancy)
	Basal and squamous cell carcinomas	Albinism I & II (congenital absence of pigment production)
	Ileum adenocarcinoma	Cystic fibrosis (chronic lung infections, pancreatic insufficiency)
	Sarcomas	Werner syndrome (multi-system problems related to premature aging)
	Hepatocellular carcinoma	Hemochromatosis (iron storage disorder)
X-Linked	Lymphoma	X-linked lymphoproliferative syndrome
	Squamous cell cancers and pancreatic adenocarcinoma	Dyskeratosis congenita (leucoplakia, nail dystrophy, DD, pigmentation)
Chromosomal	Leukemia	Down syndrome (trisomy 21)
	Gonadoblastoma	45,X/46,XY
	Breast and testicular cancer	Klinefelter syndrome (XXY) (tall, female body habitus, small testes, infertility)
	Chondrosarcoma	Langer–Gideon syndrome (deletion 8q24.13) (DD, microcephaly, characteristic facial features with scant, fragile hair, multiple exostoses and other skeletal anomalies)

[a]DD = developmental delay.
Sources: Friedman (1997); Gorlin et al., (1990); NCI (1996); Offit (1998); Vogelstein and Kinzler (1998).

type of juvenile polyposis syndrome may actually have a missed diagnosis of Cowden syndrome (or they may develop symptoms with aging) (Eng and Ji, 1998; Howe et al., 1998).

For the patient interested in cancer genetic counseling, a family pedigree can be quite expansive, often extending *five* generations! Take the example of Leanne, a 32-year-old mother of three young daughters who is anxious about her chances of developing cancer. Beatrice, Leanne's 60-year-old mother, survived breast cancer diagnosed at age 42 years, but now Beatrice has a newly diagnosed ovarian cancer. At a minimum you would inquire about any cancers in Beatrice's parents and grandparents, her aunts and uncles, her siblings, her nieces and nephews, and her children and grandchildren. On the pedigree it is just as important to note which family members have cancer as to record who is *unaffected*. When a relative with cancer is identified, the medical-family history should extend as far back in prior generations as possible. Information about the health of the children and grandchildren of affected relatives is also important. Remember to inquire about any family history of cancer in the *spouse* of an affected relative. It is easy to forget that breast-ovarian cancer syndromes can be inherited through a healthy male relative.

Paramount to accurate genetic risk assessment is the correct notation of the age of onset of cancer(s) and the type of primary cancer(s). The medical information relayed by the consultand regarding cancers in family members can be alarmingly inaccurate, particularly when recalling information about deceased relatives and family members who are related as second degree relatives or beyond (Breuer et al., 1993; Theis et al., 1994; Kerber and Slattery, 1997; Schneider et al., 1997). In a study by Love and colleagues (1985), the tumor histology verified the reported medical history of cancer in 83% of first-degree relatives (i.e., parents, siblings, children), but only 60% of second-degree relatives (i.e., grandparents, aunts and uncles, half-siblings, nieces and nephews, grandchildren), and 67% of third-degree relatives (i.e., cousins). A Utah study observed higher sensitivity for the subjects' reports of breast (83%), colorectal (73%), and prostate (70%) cancers, but less precise recall of ovarian (60%) and uterine (30%) cancers (Kerber and Slattery, 1997). A 14% error corroborating family history information with clinical data was found in a study of ovarian cancer in Alberta, Canada (Kock et al., 1989). Errors included missed malignancies, benign lesions graded as malignancies, and incorrect cancer site as well as inaccurate dates of birth, diagnosis, and death. Kerr and colleagues (1998) describe five families seen in a family cancer clinic where a factitious family or personal history led to an erroneous risk estimation.

Some common errors patients make in recalling cancer events in a family history include:

- The relative providing family history information may not make a distinction between multiple sites of primary cancers and metastatic disease. For example, the brain is a common site of metastasis for breast, melanoma, lung, kidney, and gastrointestinal cancers (National Cancer Institute, 1996). Many people will mistakenly report that Grandma had breast cancer and then brain cancer, when it was actually breast cancer metastasized to the brain (refer to Table 5.6).

TABLE 5.6   Preferential Metastatic Sites of Some Human Tumors

Primary Tumor	Common Distant Site(s)
Breast adenocarcinoma	Bone, lung, liver, brain, adrenal
Prostate adenocarcinoma	Bone
Lung small cell carcinoma	Bone, brain, liver
Skin cutaneous melanoma	Brain, liver, bowel
Thyroid adenocarcinoma	Bone
Kidney clear cell carcinoma	Bone, liver, thyroid
Testis carcinoma	Liver
Bladder carcinoma	Brain
Neuroblastoma	Liver, adrenal

Source: Reprinted from Moghaddam and Bicknell (1995), p. 48, with permission from John Wiley & Sons, Ltd.

- Family members may be embarrassed to discuss "personal cancers." For example, ovarian or uterine cancer may be referred to as a "female cancer," or someone may fail to make a distinction between testicular cancer and prostate cancer.
- Women with several affected relatives with breast cancer may over-report the number of people with breast cancer (Parent et al., 1997). For example, the historian may believe a relative had breast cancer when actually a biopsy was benign.
- Melanoma is easily confused with basal and squamous cell carcinomas (Aitken et al., 1996)
- Medical information on common cancers (such as breast and colon) is more likely to be correct than on rare cancers (e.g., osteosarcomas) (Schneider et al., 1997)

Suggestions for strategies to assist families in obtaining medical documentation of tumor pathology are discussed in Chapter 6. Information on death certificates can also be useful as a way of determining the types of cancer affecting relatives (See Chapter 6). There are common organ sites for metastasis of some human tumors as noted in Table 5.6. In taking a family history, if you are unable to obtain reports of tumor pathology, an awareness of these preferential metastatic sites may sway your index of suspicion in the direction of a metastatic process versus concluding that an individual had multiple primaries.

Noting the sex of *all* individuals on the pedigree, both affected and *unaffected,* is essential. A tumor site may be sex-limited, potentially masking the autosomal dominant pattern of disease expression. It is unusual for a man to have breast cancer but a healthy father can pass a gene alteration for breast/ovarian cancer susceptibility to his children. A hereditary prostate cancer may be difficult to recognize if a man with prostate cancer has several sisters and no brothers. If a woman has a history of premenopausal breast cancer, it just as important to document how many female relatives did *not* have breast cancer, as it is to document the relatives with cancer in the family. If a man with prostate cancer has five healthy brothers you may have fewer concerns that he has an inherited prostate cancer.

The cancers in familial cancer syndromes tend to occur at an earlier age than usual. In the breast-ovarian cancer syndromes, breast cancer is often pre-menopausal. The age of onset of colon cancer in familial adenomatous polyposis (FAP) and hereditary non-polyposis colorectal cancer (HNPCC) tends to be before age 50. Li–Fraumeni syndrome is partially characterized by childhood cancers, particularly sarcomas and adrenocortical carcinoma. Early studies on hereditary prostate cancer suggest that the age of onset of the hereditary forms are more likely to be before the ages of 50–60 years (Gronberg et al., 1997; Gail Jarvik, personal communication). It is important to note the age (ideally the date and year of birth) of both affected and unaffected individuals.

Potential environmental and occupational risk factors should be recorded in a cancer family history (Table 5.7). For example, lung cancer in a 70-year-old man with a 50-pack-year history of smoking is not surprising, but lung cancer in a 30-year-old nonsmoker is remarkable. (A pack-year is defined as smoking 20 cigarettes

TABLE 5.7   Life-style and Occupational Risk Factors for Cancer

Exposure	Related Cancer
Tobacco smoking	Mouth, pharynx, larynx, lung, esophagus, stomach, pancreas, kidney, bladder
Alcohol	Breast, colon, mouth, pharynx, larynx, esophagus, liver
Dietary fats	Possible association with colon, prostate, lung, breast
Red meat consumption	Colon
Betel nut chewing	Mouth
Sun exposure	Skin cancer
Multiple sexual partners	Cervix
Arsenic (mining, pesticides)	Lung, liver, skin
Asbestos (shipyard, mining, cement, millers, textile, pipe insulation)	Lung, larynx, mesothelioma
Aromatic amines (dyes)	Bladder
Benzene (varnishes, other industrial uses)	Leukemia
Bis-ether	Lung
Shoe manufacturing	Nasal cavity
Chromium (metal plating)	Lung
Hardwood manufacturing	Nasal cavity
Hematite mining	Lung
Isopropyl alcohol manufacturing	Para-nasal sinuses
Mustard gas	Lung, pharynx, larynx
Nickel refining	Lung, nasal sinuses
Rubber industry (benzidine, napthylamine)	Leukemia, bladder
Soots, tars, oils	Skin, lung, bladder
Vinyl chloride (PVC)	Liver (angiosarcoma)

Sources: Revised from Offit (1998) p. 34, and reprinted with permission from John Wiley and Sons, Inc. Other source: National Cancer Institute (1996).

a day for a year. A person who smokes two packs of cigarettes a day for 10 years has a 20 pack-year history of tobacco smoking.) Increasingly, viruses are being linked to human cancers (National Cancer Institute, 1996; Offit, 1998):

- Human papilloma virus with cervical and squamous cell carcinomas
- Hepatitis B and C with hepatic carcinoma
- HTLV1 (human lymphotropic virus 1) with adult T-cell leukemia/lymphoma
- Epstein Barr virus with nasopharyngeal carcinoma, Burkitt's lymphoma and post-transplantation polycolonal lymphomas, Kaposi's sarcoma, and lymphomas
- HIV infection with Kaposi's sarcoma, and non-Hodgkins lymphoma

Recording the ethnicity of family members is significant because a number of "founder" mutations have been identified (Szabo and King, 1997; Laken et al., 1997). For example, in Iceland there is a common breast cancer mutation in BRCA2 called 999del5. There are two mutations in the BRCA1 gene (185delAG and 5382insC) and one mutation in BRCA2 (6174delT) that are common in the Ashkenazi Jewish population (Offitt, 1998).

SUMMARY

The instruments of molecular genetics, in concert with a precise genetic family history, provide clinicians with powerful investigative tools to identify individuals with an increased risk to develop various cancers. With the ever-expanding palette of commercially available tests that predict cancer susceptibility, medical professionals must be prepared to offer accurate counseling about the meaning of a positive, negative, or ambiguous test result. Testing, if performed, must be interpreted in the context of the family history. Such testing, done poorly, can cause far more harm than benefit. Test results can have profound reverberations for an individual's psychological and physical health, insurability, as well as family and social functioning (Greely, 1997; McKinnon et al., 1997; Schneider, 1994). Cautions Dr. Kenneth Offit (1998), Chair of the American Society of Clinical Oncology's Subcommittee on Genetic Testing for Cancer Susceptibility, "A genetic test of outstanding scientific interest is of little clinical value if the clinician is unable to interpret it, the patient afraid or unsure how to act on it, and the national health-care system unable to provide it without penalty or discrimination."

A dramatic example of the power of pedigree analysis is shown in Figure 5.1. A healthy 29-year-old woman is concerned about her risk to develop breast cancer given a history of breast cancer in her mother and maternal aunt, with no other family history of breast or other cancers. The occurrence of postmenopausal breast cancer in her aunt and mother does not significantly change her risk to develop breast cancer from that of other women her age. In contrast, the consultand's lifetime risk to develop breast cancer (based on empirical risk figures from the Claus model) ap-

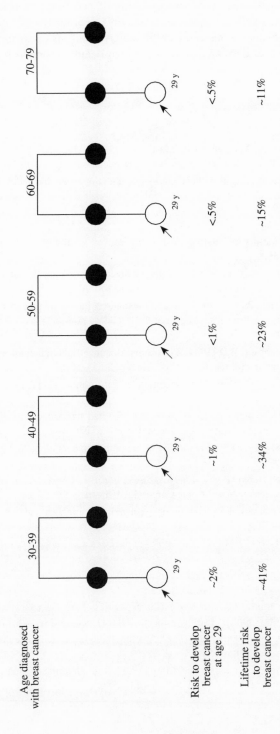

Figure 5.1 The empirical risk to develop breast cancer based on the age of onset of breast cancer in a mother and maternal aunt. Note that that if the consultand's mother and aunt develop breast cancer between the ages of 70 and 79 years, the consultand's lifetime risk to develop breast cancer is the same as any woman's lifetime risk to develop cancer by age 80. Risk figures derived from Claus et al., 1994.

proaches that of an autosomal dominant syndrome if her mother and aunt have breast cancer diagnosed in their 30s (Claus et al., 1994). For many individuals with fears about a family history of cancer, careful pedigree analysis can reassure them that their lifetime risk to develop cancer is not significantly different from other people their age.

REFERENCES

Aitken JF, Youl P, Green A, MacLennan R, Martin NG (1996). Accuracy of case-reported family history of melanoma in Queensland, Australia. Melanoma Res 6(4):313–317.

Akiyama Y, Sato H, Yamada T, et al. (1997). Germ-line mutation of the hMSH6/GTBP gene in an atypical hereditary nonpolyposis colorectal cancer kindred. Cancer Res. 57:3920–3923.

Breuer B, Kash KM, Rosenthal G, Diemer K, Osborne MP, Miller DG (1993). Reporting bilaterality status in first-degree relatives with breast cancer: a validity study. Genet Epidemiol 10(4):245–256.

Burke W, Daly M, Garber J, et al. (1997). Recommendations for follow-up care of individuals with an inherited predisposition to cancer: BRCA1 and BRCA2. JAMA 277:997–1003.

Burke W, Petersen G, Lynch P, et al. (1997). Recommendations for follow-up care of individuals with an inherited predisposition to cancer: I. Hereditary non-polyposis colon cancer. JAMA 277:915–919.

Claus EB, Risch N, Thompson WD (1994). Autosomal dominant inheritance of early-onset breast cancer. Implications for risk prediction. Cancer 73:643–651.

Cummings S, Olufunmilayo O (1998). Predisposition testing for inherited breast cancer. Oncology: 1227–1242.

Eng C, Ji H (1998). Molecular classification of the inherited hamartoma polyposis syndromes: clearing the muddied waters. Am J Hum Genet 62:1020–1022.

Flanders TY, Foulkes WD (1996). Pancreatic adenocarcinoma: epidemiology and genetics, J Med Genet 33:889–898.

Foulkes WD, Hodgson SV (eds) (1998). *Inherited Susceptibility to Cancer: Clinical, Predictive and Ethical Perspectives.* Cambridge: Cambridge University Press.

Friedman JM (1997). Genetics and epidemiology, congenital anomalies and cancer. Am J Hum Genet 60:469–473.

Gorlin RJ, Cohen MM, Levin LS (1990). *Syndromes of the Head and Neck.* New York:Oxford University Press.

Greely HT (1997). Genetic testing for cancer susceptibility: challenges for creators of practice guidelines. Oncology 11:171–176.

Gronberg H, Issacs SD, Smith JR, et al. (1997). Characteristics of prostate cancer in families potentially linked to the hereditary prostate cancer 1 (HPC1) locus. JAMA 278:1251–1255.

Hemminki A, Markie D, Tomlinson, et al. (1998). A serine/threonine kinase gene defective in Peutz–Jeghers syndrome. Nature 391:184–187.

Hisada M, Garber JE, Fung CY, Fraumeni JF, Li FP (1998). Multiple primary cancers in families with Li–Fraumeni syndrome. JNCI 90:606–611.

Howe JR, Ringold JC, Summers RW, et al. (1998). A gene for familial juvenile polyposis maps to chromosome 18q21.1. Am J Hum Genet 62:1129–1136.

Jacoby RF, Schlack S, Sekhon G, Laxova R (1997). Del (10)(q22.3q24.1) associated with juvenile polyposis. Am J Med Genet 70:361–364.

Jenne DE, Reimann H, Nezu J, et al. (1998). Peutz-Jeghers syndrome is caused by mutations in a novel serine threonine kinase. Nature Genet 18:38–43.

Kerber RA, Slattery ML (1997). Comparison of self-reported and database-linked family history of cancer data in a case-control study. Am J Epidemiol 146(3):244–248.

Kerr B, Foulkes WD, Cade D et al. (1998). False family history in the family cancer clinic. Euro J Surg Onc 24:275–279.

Kock M, Gaedke H, Jenkins H (1989). Family history of ovarian cancer patients: a case-control study. Int J Epidemiol 18:782–785.

Laken SJ, Petersen G, Gruber S, et al. (1997). An APC mutation associated with familial colorectal cancer in Ashkenazi Jews. Nature Genet 17:79–83.

Liaw D. Marsh DJ, Li J, et al. (1997). Germline mutations of the PTEN gene in Cowden disease, an inherited breast and thyroid cancer syndrome. Nature Genet 16:64–67.

Love R, Evans AM, Josten DM (1985). The accuracy of patient reports of a family history of cancer. J Chron Dis 38:289–293.

Lynch ED, Ostermeyer EA, Lee MK, et al. (1997). Inherited mutations that are associated with breast cancer, Cowden disease, and juvenile polyposis. Am J Hum Genet 61:1254–1260.

Lynch HT, Fusaro RM, Lynch JF (1997). Cancer genetics in the new era of molecular biology. Ann NY Acad Sci :1–27.

Marsh DJ, Dahia PLM, Zheng Z et al. (1997). Germline mutations in PTEN are present in Bannayan-Zonana syndrome. Nature Genet 16:333–334.

McKinnon WC, Baty B, Bennett RL, et al. (1997). Predisposition genetic testing for late-onset disorders in adults: a points to consider document of the National Society of Genetic Counselors. JAMA 278:1217–1220.

Mehenni H, Blouin JL, RadhakrishnaV, et al. (1997). Peutz-Jeghers syndrome: confirmation of linkage to chromosome 1p13.3 and identification of a potential second locus on 19q 13.4. Am J Hum Genet 61:1327–1334.

Miyaki M, Konishi M, Tanaka K, et al. (1997). Germline mutation of MSH6 as the cause of hereditary nonpolyposis colorectal cancer. Nature Genetics 17:271–272.

Moghaddam A, Bicknell R (1995). The organ preference of metastasis—The journey from the circulation to secondary site. In Vile RG (ed), *Cancer Metastasis: From Mechanisms to Therapies.* New York: John Wiley & Sons, p. 48.

National Cancer Institute (1996). *Cancer Rates and Risks.* National Institutes of Health.

Offit K (1998). *Clinical Cancer Genetics: Risk Counseling and Management.* New York: John Wiley & Sons.

Olschwang S, Serova-Sinilnikova OM, Lenoir GM, Thomas G (1998). PTEN germ-line mutations in juvenile polyposis coli [letter]. Nat Genet 18:12–14.

Parent ME, Ghadirian P, Lacroix A, Perret C (1997). The reliability of recollections of family history: implications for the medical provider. J Cancer Education 12(2):114–120.

Schmidt L, Fuh-Mei D, Chen F, et al. (1997). Germline and somatic mutations in the tyrosine kinase domain of the MET proto-oncogene in papillary renal carcinomas. Nature Genet 16:68–73.

Schneider KA (1994). *Counseling About Cancer: Strategies for Genetic Counselors.* Available from Dana-Farber Cancer Institute, Div. Cancer Epidemiology & Control, 44 Binney St., 3A Mayer, Boston, MA 02115.

Schneider K, Patenaude A, DiGianni L, Garber J (1997). Accuracy in reporting family histories of cancer among participants in a P53 testing program. J Genet Counsel 6(4):A509–510.

Spitz JL (1996). *Genodermatoses. A Full-Color Clinical Guide to Genetic Skin Disorders.* Baltimore: Williams & Wilkin.

Szabo CI, King MC (1997). Population genetics of BRCA1 and BRCA2. Am J Hum Genet 60:1013–1020.

Theis B, Boyd N, Lockwood G, Tritchler D (1994). Accuracy of family cancer history in breast cancer patients. Eur J Cancer Prev 3(4):321–327.

Vogelstein B, Kinzler KW (eds) (1998). *The Genetic Basis of Human Cancer.* New York: McGraw-Hill.

Williams TT (1991). *Refuge, An Unnatural History of Family and Place.* New York: Vintage Books.

6

Medical Verification of a Family History

There is a moral and philosophical respect for our ancestors,
which elevates the character and improves the heart.
—Daniel Webster

VALIDATION OF FAMILY MEDICAL INFORMATION IS AN ABSOLUTE NECESSITY

Genetic diseases are unique in that a whole family is, in essence, your patient. Confirming family rhetoric by obtaining medical records may be time consuming, but it is essential. Two glaring illustrations from my own practice emphasize the need to corroborate oral reports of family-medical history information with formal medical documentation:

1. "Elizabeth," a healthy 40-year-old woman, requested presymptomatic testing for Huntington disease (an autosomal dominant, adult-onset, neurodegenerative condition). Her father and sister reportedly died of complications from Huntington disease. Although accurate DNA testing is available to identify the gene mutation in Huntington disease, we insisted that Elizabeth obtain her father's and sister's medical records to confirm their diagnoses. Our perusal of these medical records suggested her father and sister had a similar neurodegenerative illness, though the symptoms were not typical of Huntington disease. We arranged for additional neuropathology studies on the stored brain tissue from her sister's autopsy, and actually diagnosed a form of autosomal dominant cerebellar ataxia. If Elizabeth had proceeded with DNA testing for Huntington disease, her testing would have been nor-

mal. Elizabeth would have been falsely reassured that she was no longer at risk for her family's devastating neurodegenerative illness, when in fact she remained at 50:50 risk to develop the same disease that affected her father and sister. Given this new information we were able to offer Elizabeth appropriate genetic counseling with the option for accurate genetic testing.

2. "Diane," a healthy 30-year-old woman, was interested in information about her risks to develop ovarian cancer; her mother apparently had died of ovarian cancer 8 years ago at age 50 years. Aside from the history that Diane's 70-year-old maternal uncle died of stomach cancer, there was no other family history of cancer. We obtained pathology reports on the tumors in both of these individuals; Diane's mother did not have ovarian cancer but actually metastatic cancer to her abdomen of unknown primary origin (*not* believed to be ovarian), and Diane's uncle had metastatic melanoma. Diane was planning to have an oophorectomy because of her overwhelming fear of ovarian cancer. We were able to reassure Diane that we did not recognize an obvious hereditary cancer syndrome in her family, and that she should be screened for cancer in the same manner as any other woman her age. She cancelled her surgery.

Most people have limited information about the details of the medical health of their extended family. Your patient may know that his father and paternal grandfather died of colon cancer, but he is unlikely to know the details from the pathology reports. Even the "family genealogist" may know few medical details about family members. The traditions of genealogy focus on recording dates and locations of significant kinship alliances (such as births, deaths, and marriages), but not documenting family illness. In fact, the purpose of early pedigrees was to document kinships for creating alliances of land and wealth, as well as to prove relationship to aristocracy.

Although the onus is on your patient to obtain medical and family history information, your patient may be at a total loss as to where and how to begin. Such a task may seem especially daunting if the patient is physically or emotionally distanced from the family. This chapter contains several resources for your patients to help them approach family members to obtain further medical history information. I have also included resources for patients to learn how to record their own family pedigree. This information is meant to encourage patients to be partners in their health care.

HOW TO APPROACH FAMILY MEMBERS

These days there is a wondrous array of methods for communication. A patient may choose to initiate contact with family members by telephone, letter, FAX, or E-mail. Several Internet search engines can comb the "White Pages" for the phone numbers, E-mail, and mailing addresses of forgotten relatives. I find Yahoo People Search (URL: http://www.four11.com) a particularly useful web site for this purpose. Often the most effective means of approaching family members about obtaining medical and family history data is in person, at a family gathering.

Family members who fear an invasion of privacy may feel better about sharing the intimate details of their medical lives if only specific information is requested as compared to a blanket request to browse their medical records. Aunt Martha may be willing to share the pathology report from her breast surgery, but not the entire account of her painful emotional and physical recovery from a radical mastectomy.

THE PRIVACY OF A PERSON'S LIFE

Medical records contain more than just medical facts. The records may reveal family secrets such as adoption, false paternity, mental instability, sexual orientation, or drug and alcohol abuse. Records, which seem "dry" to a health professional, may be charged with emotions for the relative who reads them. An adult may be reminded of the trauma of losing a mother to breast cancer (Matloff, 1997). The records may chronicle the short, medically involved life of a much-desired child who died of a severe chromosome anomaly. In researching my own medical-family history I obtained the account of my grandfather's tumultuous death from pancreatic cancer. Although he died years before my birth, I felt awkward knowing the intimacies of the last breaths of life of this man I never met. When a patient requests sensitive family medical records, I often warn him or her to open this mail at a time when there is an opportunity for reflection.

REQUESTING MEDICAL DOCUMENTATION

The most efficacious way to obtain medical records is to provide your patient with your medical center's official consent form for requesting medical information. The patient takes the responsibility to sends the release form(s) to the appropriate family member(s), who in turn sends signed release forms to the appropriate medical facility. The medical records are then sent directly to your office. If the inquiry is via a health professional there is often no charge to the patient for gathering medical records. Private physician offices and small medical centers may charge fees in the range of $10–$25 for this service. Table 6.1 provides a sample letter to accompany the release form instructing a family member on how to fill out the medical consent form. I try to be as explicit as possible in requesting information. As shown in Figure 6.1, I complete the top of the release form with my address and phone number, and specify the types of medical information I am looking for. Depending on the disease, I anticipate the medical records that *might* be available, and I request documentation accordingly. For example:

- Muscle biopsy findings, creatine kinase levels, electromyogram, and DNA test results for a relative with a reported muscular dystrophy
- Pathology and surgical reports for a relative with cancer

TABLE 6.1   Sample Letter to Request a Family Member's Medical Records

Date:

Relative's or Patient's Name and Address

Dear_____:

Enclosed you will find "consent to obtain information" forms. These release forms give us permission to obtain your medical records or medical records from a family member. We need this information for your medical appointment. All information obtained will be confidential.

The release form should be sent directly to the appropriate hospital, physician, or agency. They will forward the records directly to us.

The consent form should be signed by the person (or his/her legal guardian or next-of kin) whose medical information is being obtained. If the consent form is signed by anyone other than the patient, please note the relationship (e.g., daughter—closest surviving next-of-kin, or mother—legal guardian). To assist the Medical Records Department, print or type the full name (first, middle, and all last names, including maiden name), and the birth date (write out the name of the month). If the person is deceased, include the date and year of death. Include approximate dates of treatment or hospitalization at the medical facility (e.g., January 1988, 1960–1967, etc.). Include the person's social security number if you know this information (especially if the medical records are being requested from a military medical facility).

If you have any questions about these forms or about your appointment, please call me at _____. Thank you for your help in obtaining the information we need.

Sincerely,

Name of Health Care Provider or Office Manager

- Neurodevelopmental testing, metabolic screening, chromosome analysis, and brain imaging studies for a child with a progressive mental retardation
- Birth records, intensive care notes, and autopsy records for a child born with multiple congenital anomalies who died soon after birth

In hopes of getting as much information as possible on deceased family members, I request autopsy information even if my patient is not sure if one was performed. I highlight, or mark with a large red X, the sections of the release form the patient must complete.

It is best to provide the Medical Records Department with as much identifying information on the relative as possible. Names should include the first, middle, and last names, all surnames (including maiden names), aliases, and designations such as "Junior," "Senior," "II," or "III." Provide complete birth dates (spell out the months so there is no confusion between abbreviations for date or month of birth). Social security numbers are useful (and essential if you are obtaining records that are from a military facility).

Please Return One Copy of This Form with Your Report To:

Attention: *(Your name and phone number)*

           (Name)   (Dept)   (Phone)

BEST HOSPITAL
0000 Good Health St.
Anywhere, WA 99999-9999

TO: Name   *(Fill this out for patient, if known)*

            Address _____

            City/State/Zip _____

The below-named patient or his/her authorized representative request you furnish **Best Hospital** with the information listed below. This information would be of great value in expediting the patient's medical assessment

_____ **INFORMATION TO BE DISCLOSED** _____

Please Check all Appropriate Boxes

☑ Summary of Medical History/Treatment   ☑ Radiology Records *brain CT/MRI*

☑ Laboratory/Diagnostic Tests *genetic, metabolic*   ❑ Radiology Films_____

❑ All Records, including any records in these subject areas:

❑ HIV/AIDS   ❑ Drug and Alcohol Abuse

❑ Sexually Transmitted Disease   Treatment

❑ Mental Illness or Mental Health Treatment

☑ OTHER: *evaluations for developmental delay, genetic studies, chromosomes*

The purpose of the disclosure: *coordination of care*

State and federal law protect information disclosed by this consent. These laws prohibit making any further disclosure of this information without the specific written consent of the person to whom it pertains, or as otherwise permitted by state law. This consent is subject to revocation at any time except to the extent that the program that is to make the disclosure has already taken action in reliance on it. This consent expires on _____ or in (90) days unless otherwise specified.

_____ **CONSENT** _____

I hereby request the above named doctor or institution furnish Best Hospital with all information designated above from its records of:

Name under which patient was treated (please print)	Birthdate
X	X
Approximate dates of treatment and/or hospitalization X	
Date X	Signature (patient or person authorized to give consent)
If signed by person other than patient, provide reason and relationship to patient X	
Date X	Witness

Patient #:

Name: *(Your patient's name)*   **BEST HOSPITAL LOGO**

DOB:
Note relationship (e.g. nephew, maternal aunt)

Figure 6.1 *An example of how to fill out a consent form to obtain medical records on a patient or family member. Be as specific as possible as to the type of records you are requesting, and remember to note on the form how the relative is related to your patient.*

Obviously a living family member must sign for the release of his or her own medical records. For a person considered mentally incompetent, the legal guardian signs for the records. Some medical records departments require proof of guardianship papers before releasing records. The legal next-of-kin signs for a deceased individual. The order of legal next-of-kin is usually first, the surviving spouse (if married at time of death), followed by the children or parents, and then grandchildren. Siblings can usually obtain records of their deceased brother or sister if the deceased sibling does not have a surviving spouse or offspring. Nieces and nephews of a deceased relative may also be able to obtain medical records if they are the closest surviving next-of-kin. Some medical records departments require a copy of the death certificate to accompany the request for records. Persons requesting records should sign the consent form, and state their relationship to the deceased and that they are the closest surviving next-of-kin (i.e., John Hancock, grandson, closest surviving next-of-kin).

If you are obtaining medical records on several people in a family, it can be crazier than following the plot of a soap opera to keep track of family names. Before I send a consent form to my patient for distribution to the relatives, I always note at the bottom of the page how the relative is related to my patient (e.g., Darwin, Erasmus—grandfather of Darwin, Charles) (see Figure 6.1). Such a tracking method is particularly helpful when family members have the same first and last names. I also keep a copy of all release requests, and note the date the release was sent to the patient or family members. This serves as a reminder for me to contact the family again in a month or so if I have not received the requested records.

I use the *American Hospital Association (AHA) Guide to the Health Care Field* almost daily in helping my patients obtain medical records. This directory lists alphabetically all the hospitals in the United States and government hospitals abroad, as well as sorting hospitals by city and state. Your patient might know that a deceased relative was seen in a small community hospital in Yakima, Washington, but not know the facility's name and address. With this directory you can easily provide the patient with the names and addresses of all the medical facilities in that community. Your patient can then send medical release forms to all the hospitals in that community. The worst that can happen is the receipt of a return letter stating the relative did not receive medical care at that facility. The AHA Guide is produced annually and is available at a cost of approximately $95 (nonmember price $250) from AHA, One North Franklin, Chicago, IL 60606-3401 (telephone: 1-800-AHA-2626).

The information on death certificates can be notoriously inaccurate (Messite and Stellman, 1996; Magrane et al., 1997). However, the cause of death listed on a death certificate may be the only medical documentation available on a relative. VitalChek Network has a Web site (URL: http://www.vitalchek.com/) that lists contact information (FAX, E-mail, and phone) for obtaining vital records (birth and death certificates and marriage licenses) in each state. There is a small charge for obtaining vital records (the fees are listed on the Web site). VitalChek also has a toll free telephone number (800-255-2414).

EMPOWERING YOUR PATIENTS WITH TOOLS FOR RECORDING THEIR OWN MEDICAL-FAMILY HISTORIES

Your ability to provide accurate genetic assessment and genetic diagnostic testing is facilitated if a patient arrives with accurate family history information in hand. Here are some suggestions for resources to help your clients learn to collect and record the medical information on their extended families:

Growing Your Family Medical Tree (1997) by Fran Carlson. Keep It Simple Solutions, Lafayette Hill, PA 19444-0136. ~$14.95

Carlson provides a unique and fun approach to collecting medical history data by helping individuals create a "Family Deck of Life." Basic demographic and health information on each family member (living or deceased) is recorded on a 4″ × 6″ card. The "recorder" documents the "health gifts and risks" for each family member. The diseases on each card are then coded with a colored dot. For example, a green dot might represent cardiovascular disease. The color-coded cards are matched to provide clues as to patterns of health and disease in the family.

How Healthy is Your Family Tree? A Complete Guide to Tracing your Family's Medical and Behavioral Tree (1995) by Carol Krause. A Fireside Book, Simon & Schuster, New York. $12.00

Krause uses her riveting personal story of her own family's striking history of cancer to compel the reader to record his or her own family medical tree to "save your life." This is an actual workbook taking the reader through a step-by-step process of how to obtain this medical information, and how to record a medical pedigree. Krause includes practical information such as sample letters on where and how to obtain death certificates, and suggestions for approaching family members for medical information. The book includes a helpful checklist of the demographic and health information needed on each ancestor, followed by the explanation as to why this information is necessary. Krause takes the workbook model a step further by guiding the reader through a "consumer friendly genogram." A genogram is a tool developed by family therapists to use symbols, in a format similar to a medical pedigree, to identify communication patterns between all family members, biological or not. A traditional genogram is usually not a useful tool in genetic assessment because medical information is often lacking (McGoldrick and Gerson, 1985). However, persons with a genetic disease in the family may benefit from the visual nature of a genogram to portray family strengths and recognize ineffective communication patterns. This process may help individuals develop coping strategies for dealing with the profound impact of a genetic condition on the entire family.

The Family Genetic Sourcebook (1990) by Benjamin Pierce. John Wiley & Sons, Inc., New York. $14.95

Although somewhat dated, this book provides good information at a reasonable price. There are four main sections to this book: (1) basic genetic principles, and a "catalogue" of genetic diseases and inherited traits; (2) information about genetic counseling; (3) step-by-step information about how to record a pedigree; and (4) resources including state-by-state contact information for clinical genetic services. This is particularly helpful for clinicians that may need to arrange genetic testing for a family member who lives in another state.

The Oxford Guide to Family History (1993) by David Hey. Oxford University Press, Oxford and New York. $39.95

Although this book does not emphasize how to collect medical health history, it is a fascinating account of how to sort through the various historical registries (e.g., parish records, estate records, census data) to research a family's history. There is a beautifully illustrated pedigree of Elizabeth I tracing her family history all the way back to Adam!

Genetic Connections: A Guide to Documenting Your Individual and Family History (1995) by Danette L. Nelson-Anderson and Cynthia V. Waters. Sonters Publishing, Washington, MO. $34.95

Nelson-Anderson and Waters provide a thorough step-by-step process for recording a medical family history. A tear-out family history form is included, with pedigree paper and a drawing template. The pedigree examples are from the recommendations of the 1995 National Society of Genetic Counselors Pedigree Standardization Task Force. The authors lead the reader through a medical systems approach to taking a family history. Most of the health conditions in the book do not have a strict genetic etiology.

Public Broadcasting Series, "Ancestors (Episode 8)—Medical Heritage" (1997), 30-minute video. $19.95

Ancestors is a multi-episode PBS series on how to research ancestral history. This episode features an interview with genetic counselor Vickie Venne and medical geneticist Dr. Raymond White, who demonstrates how to use genealogy information to draw a family medical pedigree. Interviewers Jim and Terry Willard share the emotional story of Carol Krause, a woman whose family is ravaged by cancer, as a way to convince the viewer of the importance of obtaining a family medical history.

SOFTWARE PROGRAMS FOR RECORDING FAMILY HISTORIES

Some genealogical software programs incorporate the ability to draw pedigrees (called a box chart in genealogy circles). These programs allow users to create jazzy multi-media living pedigrees, with the opportunity to synthesize medical information with family photographs and videotapes, favorite recipes, even audiotapes of family members reciting the family folklore! A listing of genealogy software programs can be found on the Ancestors homepage (see below). My current software favorites are *Ultimate Family Tree* (Palladium, for MacIntosh, $19.95–$59.95 depending on the version), *Family Tree Maker Deluxe Edition III,* v. 4.4 (Broderbund, for Windows or MacIntosh, $99.95), and *Family Origins* (Parsons Technology, Windows, $29.00).

RESOURCES FROM THE GENEALOGICAL GURUS

The Internet has opened amazing avenues for genealogical research. A few of the more informative sites include the following:

http://www.genealogy.org	Genealogy Online. A wonderful link to the searchable genealogical Web databases
http://www.worldgenweb.org	World GenWeb Project. A noncommercial project to provide genealogical searches worldwide
http://www.ancestry.com	Ancestors Home Page. Features include the Genealogy Shoppe (ideas for gifts for your favorite genealogist), and for a nominal monthly fee subscribers receive a newsletter and access to databases
http://www.census.gov	Homepage for the US Census Bureau. Contains information about how to access their publications
http://www.oz.net/~cyndihow/	Mark and Cyndi Howell's Family Tree Site. An award-winning site with over 38,850 genealogical web resources indexed in more than 90 categories
http://www.genetics.com.au/fhtg.htm	Drawing Your Family Health Tree. A Web site maintained by a genetics program in Australia. Provides information on how to construct a family pedigree incorporating standardized pedigree symbols

REFERENCES

Magrane BP, Gilliand MGF, King DE (1997). Certificates of death by family physicians. Am Fam Phy 56:1433–1438.

Matloff ET (1997). Generations lost: a cancer genetics case report. J Genet Couns 6:169-176.

McGoldrick M, Gerson R (1985). *Genograms in Family Assessment.* New York: W. W. Norton and Company.

Messite J, Stellman SD (1996). Accuracy of death certificate completion: need for family physician training. JAMA 275:794–796.

7

The Challenge of Family History and Adoption

Knowing one's ancestors is not a matter of mild curiosity; it is often part of an attempt to explain life and to understand how we have come to be what we are, not just physically through inherited genes, but how we have come to believe in certain principles or to have acquired the attitudes, prejudices, and characteristics that mould our personality. For very many people, tracing a family tree and discovering the lives of their ancestors is not a task that is undertaken lightly.
—*David Hey (1993)*

THE PROBLEM DEFINED

A thorough family history is an extremely important part of the adoption process. The lifelong medical care of an individual may be facilitated by access to health and family history information gathered at the time of adoption. Medical information in the adoption records may also be beneficial to an adult making reproductive choices. The availability of sophisticated DNA testing will not obviate the usefulness of a genetic family history, for genetic testing is done in the context of family history. This chapter is for the health professional (or the professional adoption intermediary) involved in gathering medical and family history information for a child being placed for adoption. It also includes resources for searching for information on a birth parent and trying to open sealed adoption records.

Any adoption involves a tangled web of interests, including those of the adoptive parents, the birth family, the adopted individual, and the designated intermediaries (e.g., adoption agency, attorney). The legal and emotional needs of these individuals are complex, and often at odds with each other. Adoptive parents are increasingly interested in genetic testing and family history information about their children. Yet these same parents may be ambivalent about contact with their child's biological relatives. Biological parents may be interested in information about their child's adjustment in the years following the adoption, and they often want to communicate with their adult child. In fact, there is a growing trend toward "open adoptions," where the birth mother participates in the selection of the adoptive parents. In parallel, many adopted individuals maintain a healthy curiosity about their biological ancestry, in addition to needing their biological history for medical reasons. Information about the adopted individual's biological roots may even help protect that individual from the psychological trauma of an identity crisis termed "genealogical bewilderment" (Bender, 1989). All these variables frequently lead to conflicts of interest related to the psychological welfare, medical needs, and legal rights of the parties involved in an adoption.

A HISTORICAL PERSPECTIVE ON THE LAWS GOVERNING ADOPTION

Adoption is a legal fiction. It assumes that a child's ties to biological parents can be displaced entirely by ties to adoptive parents. Social and psychological evidence suggest, however, that legal rules cannot so easily obliterate the past or prevent adoptees, as they grow older, from desiring to re-establish some links to their past
— Michael Bender (1989) §13.01[1][a]

Prior to the early 1900s, adoption in America was a relatively informal matter with few formal legal adoptions. The first adoption law was codified in Massachusetts in 1851,* and contained no requirement that adoption records should be either maintained or kept confidential (Bender, 1989). Almost 65 years later, laws were formulated in many jurisdictions to protect the adoption proceedings from public scrutiny. Such laws were enacted to shield birth mothers, as well as their children, from the shame and stigmatization of illegitimacy. A 1917 Minnesota statute[†] was the first law to reflect a concern about the privacy of birth parents by requiring that adoption records be kept confidential (Bender, 1989). As time went on, adoption proceedings became more surreptitious. By the mid 1920s, most states had statutes cloaking the adoption process in secrecy, providing for the sealing of adoption records and the issuance of a new birth certificate. All parties were denied access to these adoption records except under a judicial finding of "good cause" (Bender, 1989; Lorandos, 1996).

Birth parents and adopted individuals have challenged anonymity and secrecy in the adoption process. State legislatures have only recently responded to this criticism by enacting laws granting adopted children and their adoptive families access to appropriate health and family history information. Forty-one states currently pro-

*Massachusetts Acts of 1851, ch. 324.
[†]1917 Minnesota Laws chapter 222, p. 337.

vide, to varying extents, for the collection of medical information from birth parents and the release of this information to adoptive families (Lorandos, 1996). The impetus for changes in these laws has largely been in response to litigation related to "wrongful adoption." In this type of litigation, adoptive parents attempt to revoke adoptions after discovering genetic, mental, or physical problems in their adopted children (Lorandos, 1996; Zitter, 1987).

The American Society of Human Genetics has taken the stance that a genetic history should be included in an adopted individual's record. They assert that "every person should have the right to gain access to his or her medical record, including genetic data . . . . When medically appropriate, genetic data may be shared among the adoptive parents, biological parents and adoptees" (ASHG, 1991). Twenty-five states actually require compilation of a genetic history (Andrews, 1997).

Currently no state has an absolute open adoption record policy. Most states now require agencies or private intermediaries to compile comprehensive profiles of children and their biological parents, and to share this non-identifying information with the adoptive parents at the time of adoption (Bender, 1989). Each state has different requirements on the nature of the non-identifying information that is shared with the adoptive parents at the time of adoption. The non-identifying information generally includes:

- Basic information such as date, time, state, and county of the adopted child's birth
- The age of the biological parents at the time of placement and their general physical description (ranging from height and hair color to such subtleties as whether they are right- or left-handed)
- Race, ethnicity, and religion
- Whether termination of parental rights is voluntary or court-ordered
- The facts and circumstances related to the adoptive placement
- The age and sex of the adopted individual's biological siblings
- Medical history of the biological parents and the adopted child
- Information about the parents' educational levels, occupations, skills, and interests (including artistic and athletic abilities)

Some states, such as Alabama, have few provisions for the maintenance and disclosure of the information obtained at the time of adoption. In contrast, Arkansas requires that such information be maintained for 99 years, and upon request, these records are available to the adoptive and biological parents, as well as the adult offspring; even the descendants of a deceased adopted individual can have access to these records (Bender, 1989). Michigan's 1998 Adoption Law (Section 710.27) specifically states that the child's health and genetic history information is to be collected and maintained by the adoption agency. The law fails to state how this will be done, and whether or not any agency is mandated to monitor the collection, storage, and dissemination of this information.

Biological parents who have their parental rights involuntarily terminated may be unwilling or unavailable to provide family history information. This is a challenging situation that few of the current statutes address.

Adoption is a lifelong process. Ensuing family history data may become relevant after the adoption is finalized. Indeed, some jurisdictions allow for the continued collection of information subsequent to the adoption (Andrews, 1997; Bender, 1989). In Delaware, if the Family Court receives a report stating that a birth parent or the adopted individual has a genetically transmitted disorder or family pattern of disease, a statute requires that the Family Court instruct the agency that was involved with the adoption to conduct a diligent search for the adult adoptee, the adoptive parents of a minor adoptee, or the birth parents (Andrews, 1998). But, who decides what medical and genetic testing information is relevant to share with parties of the adoption triad in relation to their health monitoring and reproductive decision-making? What "burden of disease" is considered great enough to interject this information into the private adoption triad? How accurate must testing be to warrant disclosure of this information? This is certainly a formidable task that is difficult to regulate through legislation.

OBTAINING MEDICAL INFORMATION FROM A CLOSED ADOPTION

Opening files from a closed adoption can be next to impossible. Even obtaining non-identifying information recorded at the time of adoption is burdensome. Some states do not have a central state registry for adoptive records. The adopted individual must direct inquiries to the court or agency that supervised the placement. The information obtained in the files may be sparse and the adopted individual may need to search for medical and genetic histories directly from the biological parents. This may be difficult if consents for such disclosures are not on file. Given the mobile nature of our society, it may be difficult to locate biological parents whose surnames and residences have changed throughout the years.

There are many resources for beginning a search for a birth parent or adoption record. The availability of Web browsers to search for phone numbers and addresses is a boon to birth parents and adopted individuals searching for biological connections. Comprehensive information about such resources is available from:

> The National Adoption Information Clearinghouse (NAIC)
> 11425 Rockville Pike, Suite 410
> Rockville, MD 20852
> telephone: (301) 231-5612. Web site: http://www.calib.com/naic/

GENETIC TESTING OF CHILDREN BEING PLACED FOR ADOPTION

Few people would argue that medical information, genetic or otherwise, that has an *immediate* impact on the health of a child should be disclosed to the adoptive parents. But what about genetic testing of a healthy child for a medical condition that potentially *may* affect this person as an adolescent or an adult? Should every child being placed for adoption receive a battery of screening tests for potential genetic diseases, regardless of whether or not there is a treatment for each condition? Could failure to provide such genetic testing have repercussions for the adoption agency in the form of wrongful adoption litigation? For example, should an adoption agency test a healthy infant for the gene mutation for Huntington disease if the child has a parent affected with this disease? Huntington disease is a progressive neurological condition for which there is no cure. The symptoms of HD are unlikely to develop in this child for another 30–40 years. Is this genetic information necessary for the adoptive parents? Or, should the child be allowed to make the choice about genetic testing when he or she is an adult?

Among genetic professionals, there is general consensus that a minor should be genetically tested only if there is an obvious medical benefit to the child. Presymptomatic genetic testing for conditions with no available treatment should be postponed until the person is of legal age to make the choice of whether or not to be tested (ASHG/ACMG Report, 1995; Andrews et al., 1994; Clarke, 1998; Task Force on Genetic Testing, Holtzman and Watson, 1997). The fear is that perhaps the healthy child with a known genetic mutation will be treated differently by the parents, peers, the school system, and society. Ethicist Dr. Dorothy Wertz notes, "Testing for untreatable adult-onset disorders prior to adoption makes the child into a commodity undergoing quality control" (Wertz et al., 1994).

A MODEL MEDICAL AND GENETIC FAMILY HISTORY FORM FOR ADOPTIONS

In order to unify the medical and genetic history information collected at the time of adoption, the Education Committee of the Council of Regional Genetics Networks (CORN) developed a model genetic family history form (Appendix A.4). The form consists of a cover page containing identifying information about the birth parents, the child welfare agency, and the agency's file identification code. This identifying information remains with the agency, as specified by the state law, unless the birth parents agree to waive their right to confidentiality. Information is collected about the child's delivery and birth. A comprehensive questionnaire about the medical and genetic history of the birth mother and father is filled out at the time of termination of parental rights with the intent of sharing this information with the foster or adoptive parents.

For optimal use of this form, it is best if a professional adoption intermediary assist each birth parent in completing the questionnaire. Optimally the professional should have some familiarity with the medical and genetic conditions contained in the form. Each user of this model genetic history is encouraged to modify it to comply with local or state regulations.

Genetic counselors and medical geneticists are available to consult with adoption intermediaries about family history interpretation. To find a genetic counselor, contact the National Society of Genetic Counselors (see Chapter 9).

REFERENCES

American Society of Human Genetics (1991). American Society of Human Genetics Social Issues Committee Report on Genetics and Adoption: Points to Consider. Am J Hum Genet 48:1009–1010.

American Society of Human Genetics/American College of Medical Genetics (1995). ASHG/ACMG Report: Points to consider: ethical, legal and psychosocial implications of genetic testing in children and adolescents. Am J Hum Genet 57:1233–1241.

Andrews LB (1997). Gen-etiquette: genetic information, family relationships and adoption. In Rothstein MA (ed), *Genetic Secrets: Protecting Privacy and Confidentiality in the Genetic Era.* New Haven: Yale University Press, pp. 255–280.

Andrews LB, Fullarton JE, Holtzman NA, Motulsky AG (1994). *Assessing Genetic Risks, Implications for Health and Social Policy.* Washington, DC: National Academy Press.

Bender M (1989). Legal and social consequences, In: Hollinger JH (ed.) *Adoption Law and Practice,* Times Mirror Books, § 13.01[3], [2].

Clarke AJ (ed) (1998). *The Genetic Testing of Children.* Oxford: BIOS Scientific Publishers Ltd.

Hey D (1993). *The Oxford Guide to Family History.* Oxford and New York: Oxford University Press.

Holtzman NA, Watson MS (1997). *Promoting Safe and Effective Genetic Testing in the United States. Final Report of the Task Force on Genetic Testing.* National Institute of Health.

Lorandos DA (1996). Secrecy and genetics in adoption law and practice. Loyola Univ Chicago Law J, 27:277–320.

Wertz DC, Fanos JH, Reilly PR (1994). Genetic testing for children and adolescents, who decides? JAMA 272:875–881.

Zitter JM (1987). Annotation, action for wrongful adoption based on misrepresentation of child's mental or physical condition or parentage. 56 ALR 4th 375:277–319.

8

The Pedigree and Assisted Reproductive Technologies

GAMETE DONATION PROVIDES THE OPPORTUNITY FOR COUPLES AT HIGH RISK FOR GENETIC DISORDERS TO HAVE HEALTHY OFFSPRING

For a couple with a high risk to have children with a genetic disorder, certain assisted reproductive technologies (ART) can virtually eliminate their chance to pass the condition on to their offspring. Recognizing the inheritance pattern of the condition is essential for providing a couple with appropriate information about reproductive options. Table 8.1 compares how ART using donor sperm or donor ovum can significantly reduce the chances of having an affected child based on the pattern of inheritance and the affected status of the partner. For example, therapeutic (artificial) donor sperm insemination (TDI) is an option for a couple where the healthy male partner is at risk for an autosomal dominant condition, such as Huntington disease, as a way to eradicate his offspring's risk to develop Huntington disease. A healthy woman who carries an X-linked mutation (such as for Duchenne muscular dystrophy) may choose donor ovum as a method to conceive a healthy pregnancy rather than facing a 50:50 chance to have an affected son. Similarly a person carrying a balanced reciprocal chromosome translocation may consider donor insemination, or donor ovum transfer, to avoid his or her increased chances of having children with a chromosome rearrangement.

Therapeutic donor insemination is a reasonable option for a healthy couple at 25% risk to have a child with a condition inherited in a classic autosomal recessive pattern. Sperm donors must be screened for carrier status of the same recessive condition. Some gamete donation programs screen a donor for a few genetic disorders based on the donor's ethnic background. For example, a potential sperm donor with

TABLE 8.1   Comparisons of How Gamete Donation Using ART (Assisted Reproductive Technologies) Can Reduce the Risk for a Genetic Disease, Based on Different Inheritance Patterns and the Affected Status of the Partner

Affected Status of Partner	Inheritance Pattern of Condition	Prior Risk of an Affected Child	Risk of an Affected Child Using Gamete Donation
A. Therapeutic Donor Semen Insemination (TDI)			
Male partner affected			
Heterozygote	Autosomal dominant	50% son or daughter	Same as background
Hemizygote	X-linked trait	50% daughter, 0% son	Same as background
Homozygote	Autosomal recessive	75% son or daughter[a]	Carrier testing of donor (if available)[b]
Male partner asymptomatic carrier			
Heterozygote	Autosomal recessive	25% son or daughter[a]	Carrier testing of donor (if available) [b]
	Chromosome translocation	Depends on translocation	Same as maternal age related risk for chromosome anomalies
B. Donor Ovum			
Female partner affected			
Heterozygote	Autosomal dominant	50% son or daughter	Same as background
Homozygote	Autosomal recessive	75% son or daughter[a]	Carrier testing of sperm donor (if available)
Heteroplasmic	Mitochondrial	0–100% son or daughter	Same as background
Heterozygote	X-linked	50% son or daughter	Same as background
Female partner asymptomatic carrier			
Heterozygote	Autosomal recessive	(TDI is generally favored over donor ovum because the risk reduction is the same, the pregnancy success rate is higher with TDI, and TDI is not as expensive as donor ovum)	
	Chromosome translocation	Depends on translocation	Based on maternal age risks of egg donor

[a]Assuming that the partner is a carrier for the same autosomal recessive disease.
[b]Risk is usually slightly above background (less than 1%) but depends on availability and accuracy of carrier testing for donor.

ancestors from Northern Europe is screened for carrier status for cystic fibrosis, or for Tay–Sachs disease carrier status if he is Ashkenazi Jewish (see Table 3.3). For some autosomal recessive disorders, carrier testing may not be available or the screening test may not detect 100% of carriers. In this instance, the couple should know that there remains a chance, slightly above the background population risk, to have a child with the genetic disease in question. This is because the sperm donor may, by chance, also carry the gene mutation for the same recessive gene as the mother. Usually the couple's risk to have a child with the condition will be in the range of 0.5–1%, depending on the frequency of heterozygotes for that genetic disorder in the general population.

SCREENING GAMETE DONORS FOR INHERITED DISORDERS

Minimal guidelines for genetic screening of gamete donors were published in *Fertility and Sterility* in 1993. The recommendations give gamete donation programs leeway to individualize their genetic screening policies because there is choice about what conditions to screen donors for, and flexibility about the extent of family history information that should be collected from donors. A summary of the 1993 guidelines follows:

- A family history should be obtained on the donor, although the extent of the family history to be obtained is not given. Donors should not be used if they have a family history of a first-degree relative with a major malformation, a major Mendelian disorder, a common autosomal recessive disorder, or a chromosome abnormality (unless the donor has been adequately screened for the condition in question).

- The donor should not have a major inherited disorder. Major is defined as a "malformation that carries serious functional or cosmetic handicap." Obviously, the interpretation of what constitutes major problem is a matter of judgment.

- The donor should be screened for any autosomal recessive disorders that are prevalent in the donor's ethnic background, for which heterozygote testing is available (e.g., Tay–Sachs and Canavan disease screening for Ashkenazi Jewish individuals). Perceptions of what is a common disorder and what is a burdensome disorder are also subject to opinion.

- The donor should not have a familial disease with a major genetic component (such as hypertension). Because most common disorders have a hereditary component, this statement may eliminate most donors!

- The donor should not carry a chromosomal rearrangement. Most screening programs do not automatically karyotype the gamete donors because of the expense of a chromosome study.

- Men older than the fifth decade should not be used as donors (because of the association of new autosomal dominant mutations and advanced paternal age).

- Women 35 years and older should not be used as egg donors because of the increased risk for offspring with chromosomal aneuploidy.

Many programs collect descriptive information on the donor, such as hair color and texture, eye color, body build, skin color, and complexion, in an effort to match the donor characteristics with that of the partner. Some programs even collect "nongenetic" information on donors such as preferences for music and hobbies to help their clients make a psychological match with the donor.

With increasing availability of genetic testing and new techniques for assisting reproduction, screening protocols for gamete donors are likely to change. The Web page of The American Society for Reproductive Medicine (ASRM) has links to position statements and resources related to this fascinating and controversial field (URL: http://www.asrm.org/).

INTRACYTOPLASMIC SPERM INJECTION AND GENETIC DISEASE

Infertile men who have azoospermia or oligospermia because of either mechanical means (such as vasectomy) or congenital absence of the vas deferens (absence of the sperm duct) are increasingly turning to removal of the sperm directly from the testes, followed by intracytoplasmic sperm injection (ICSI), as a means of conceiving pregnancy. Because there are several inherited conditions associated with male infertility (see Chapter 4, Section 4.16 and Table 4.26), before utilizing ICSI these men should have a genetic evaluation. At a minimum this assessment should include:

- At least a three-generation pedigree focusing on medical history questions associated with male infertility (see Table 4.27).
- A karyotype (specifically for detection of XXY-Klinefelter syndrome, and chromosomal rearrangements).
- DNA testing for cystic fibrosis mutations including the 5 T allele (Dork et al., 1997).
- Molecular analysis using a panel of Y-probes looking for microscopic Y-deletions.

REPRESENTING GAMETE DONATION AND SURROGACY ON A PEDIGREE

When noting on a pedigree that a pregnancy (or child) was conceived through assisted means of reproduction, it is important to trace the biological heritage of the child and the birth mother. Although anonymous gamete donation has traditionally been encouraged, a blood relative may be a participant in ART. A gestational carrier (surrogate mother) may carry a pregnancy conceived with her sister's egg and her brother-in-law's sperm (thus the gestational carrier is also a maternal aunt to the fetus). An occasional altruistic mother has been a gestational carrier for a pregnancy conceived with her daughter's egg and her son-in-law's sperm. Rarely, for a lesbian couple, the birth mother may carry a pregnancy conceived with her ovum and sperm from the brother of her female partner.

The pedigree symbols in Figure 8.1 and the pedigree line definitions (refer to Fig. 3.1) can be applied to illustrate any combination of "parents" who utilize any method of ART. Some simple pedigree drawing rules for symbolizing ART include the following:

Definitions:
— Egg or sperm donor (D)
— Surrogate (S)
— If the woman is both the ovum donor and a surrogate, in the interest of genetic assessment, she will only be referred to as a donor (e.g., 4 and 5)
— The pregnancy symbol and its line of descent are positioned below the woman who is carrying the pregnancy.
— Family history can be taken on individuals, including donors, where history is known.

Possible Reproductive Scenarios		Comments
1. Sperm donor	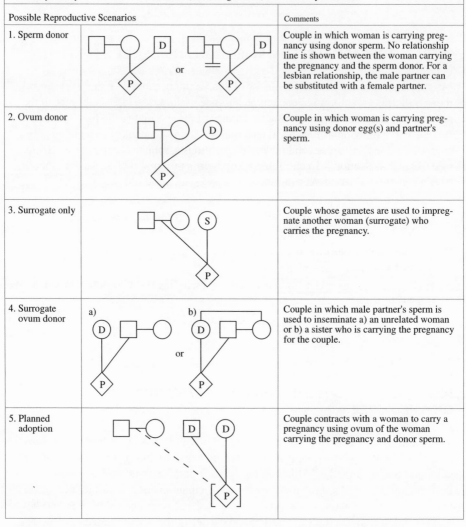	Couple in which woman is carrying pregnancy using donor sperm. No relationship line is shown between the woman carrying the pregnancy and the sperm donor. For a lesbian relationship, the male partner can be substituted with a female partner.
2. Ovum donor		Couple in which woman is carrying pregnancy using donor egg(s) and partner's sperm.
3. Surrogate only		Couple whose gametes are used to impregnate another woman (surrogate) who carries the pregnancy.
4. Surrogate ovum donor		Couple in which male partner's sperm is used to inseminate a) an unrelated woman or b) a sister who is carrying the pregnancy for the couple.
5. Planned adoption		Couple contracts with a woman to carry a pregnancy using ovum of the woman carrying the pregnancy and donor sperm.

Figure 8.1 *Pedigree symbolization of assisted reproductive technologies. Reprinted from Bennett et al., American Journal of Human Genetics (1995) with permission of the University of Chicago Press.*

- Place a "D" inside the symbol for the gamete (egg or sperm) donor.
- Place an "S" inside the female circle to represent a gestational carrier (surrogate).
- If a woman is both the ovum donor and the gestational carrier, in the interest of genetic assessment, she is referred to as a donor (thus a "D" is placed within the circle).
- The relationship line is between the couple, whether or not they are heterosexual or same-sex partners. Do not place a relationship line between the pregnant woman and the sperm donor, or between the father of the fetus (or child) and the ovum donor.
- The line of descent extends from the woman who is actually carrying the pregnancy.

SUMMARY

The methods of assisted reproductive technologies will undoubtedly continue to amaze us. By following the rules outlined in Figure 8.1, the genetic and gestational heritage of a fetus or child conceived by any imaginable assisted reproductive technology can be easily documented on a pedigree. Developing standards for screening gamete donors and gestational carriers for genetic disorders is not so easily accomplished. In putting forth such guidelines, we quickly come face to face with fundamental issues of what is a "normal" or "abnormal" human, and what is a "burdensome" inherited disease. The day that there are simple answers to these questions is the day we must question our humanity.

REFERENCES

American Fertility Society (1993). Guidelines for Gamete Donation. Fertility and Sterility 59, No. 2. Available from the American Fertility Society, 1209 Montgomery Highway, Birmingham, AL 35216.

Bennett RL, Steinhaus KA, Uhrich SB, O'Sullivan CK, Resta RG, Lochner-Doyle D, Markel DS, Vincent V, Hamanishi J (1995). Recommendations for standardized pedigree nomenclature. Am J Hum Genet 56:745–752.

Dork T, Dworniczak B, Aulehla-Scholz C, et al. (1997). Distinct spectrum of CFTR gene mutations in congenital absence of vas deferens. Hum Genet 100:365–377.

9

Making a Referral for Genetic Services: Where to Turn and What to Expect

The family had escaped the persecutions, pogroms, and poverty of Czarist Russia, but for some there would be no escape from a threat hidden within them. . . . These were days without hope. Where did it come from? How did it get started? Yet these were modern times. Why did no one know more about the disease? It was hard to believe that in this whole world our family was the only one possessing this taint. Would it ever end?
—Ben, describing his family with Alzheimer disease (Pollen, 1993)

Nothing is so soothing to our self-esteem as to find our bad traits in our forbears. It seems to absolve us.
—Van Wyck Brooks

GENETIC CONDITIONS ARE UNIQUE FROM OTHER MEDICAL CONDITIONS

Genetic information carries unique personal, family, and social consequences. Schild and Black (1984) describe six features that distinguish genetic disorders from nonhereditary medical conditions. Conditions with a genetic etiology are as follows (adapted from Costello, 1988; Plumridge et al., 1993):

1. *Familial*—Although genetic information is personal information, it could be considered "family property" because a diagnosis may embrace a whole family, not just an individual. A new genetic diagnosis in a kindred can have profound effects (both positive and negative) on interpersonal relationships among family members.

The implications of a genetic diagnosis may reverberate beyond the nuclear family, particularly if the condition is inherited in a dominant or X-linked pattern (thus placing many generations at risk). Knowledge of genetic risk factors may directly alter the reproductive plans of family members. Parental guilt is a common experience when offspring are affected with a genetic disorder. Children may blame a parent for passing on the "family curse;" offspring may bluntly query the affected parent, "Will I be like you when I grow up?" Often it is necessary to obtain medical records and even blood samples from affected family members as part of a genetic evaluation. This may be felt as an intrusion of privacy both for the person seeking the genetic information (because now other family members will know the person is involved in genetic testing) and for the family member being asked to share confidential medical and family information.

2. *Permanent*—Durable cures such as gene therapy are slow to become reality. There may be complicated management strategies such as enzyme replacement therapy for Gaucher disease, a stringent lifetime diet to prevent the mental retardation associated with phenylketonuria, or multiple surgical repairs for a deforming birth defect. There can be a sense of fatalism or hopelessness that the individual cannot "alter destiny" because the gene alteration is "in every cell of my body."

3. *Chronic*—Genetic diseases often affect individuals in different ways throughout their lifetimes. This may create chronic strains on the individual or family. Depending on the severity of the disease, the family may experience "chronic sorrow" for the person who "will never be" (Olshansky, 1962). Many individuals become increasingly impaired by their genetic condition as they age.

4. *Complex*—Genetic conditions often affect multiple organ systems. People with these conditions usually require the medical expertise of a variety of health professionals. Individuals may need unusual medical tests that are available only at major metropolitan medical centers. Patients with rare genetic disorders often meet with continual frustration trying to find health professionals that are familiar with their disorder. The rarity of the condition may give the patient and family a sense of isolation. The variable clinical expression of many genetic conditions adds to their complexity; two people with the same gene alteration may have extremely different phenotypes, making prognostic predictions difficult.

5. *Labeling*—As a society we are quick to label. A child with Down syndrome becomes "a Downs," a person with diabetes becomes "a diabetic." With a genetic label the person may perceive himself or herself as being "different, "flawed," or "mutated." The individual (and family) may have trouble with this "new identity" and grieve for his or her "former self." Family members and society may stigmatize the individual in blatant or subtle ways. For example, a person with a genetic condition might be considered less desirable as a marriage partner or as a candidate for certain employment opportunities.

6. *Threatening*—Genetic disorders threaten at many different levels including the choice of a mate, reproductive planning, privacy, self-esteem, and even longevity. The affected or at-risk individual (and his or her family) may alter long-range plans if facing a degenerative disease or premature death. The life-style of the individual and

TABLE 9.1   Common Medical Conditions with Onset in
Adulthood for Which Genetic Susceptibility Testing is
Potentially Available

Ataxia
Breast cancer
Cardiomyopathies
Colon cancer
Coronary artery disease
Dementia
Diabetes
Iron storage disease
Melanoma
Ovarian cancer
Prostate cancer

family unit may be threatened. Parents of a newborn with a severely handicapping and/or life threatening condition may have trouble bonding with the child.

If Schild and Black were writing today they would be challenged to add to the above list the phenomenon of the "unpatient" as another unique attribute of some hereditary conditions. Jonsen and colleagues (1996) coined the term "unpatients" in reference to a new-sprung category of persons who are outwardly robust but "genetically unwell;" they have inherited a gene mutation that predisposes them to develop a particular disease. It is now possible for an entirely healthy person to choose to undergo genetic testing for a cascading array of diseases that confer susceptibility to adult-onset disorders (see Table 9.1). These genetic tests cannot predict a precise age of onset of symptoms, nor can they predict the specific manifestations of disease for a particular patient. Uncertainty will probably always be a pitfall of genetic susceptibility testing. For conditions with low penetrance, individuals with the gene mutation may never develop symptoms. Additionally, a therapeutic gap exists for many of these diseases; the technical ability to test has occurred long before the availability of any effective therapy. The long-term psychological fallout of making a healthy individual "unwell" is just beginning to be explored.

WHAT IS GENETIC COUNSELING?

Genetic counseling is important because genetic disorders can affect so many areas of a person's psychological, medical, financial, and social life. Genetic counseling encompasses more than reproductive counseling about inherited disorders. Genetic counseling* is a communication process that translates technical and complicated

---

*Adapted from the definition of genetic counseling adopted by the American Society of Human Genetics in 1975.

genetic facts into practical information for individuals and families. It focuses on the human problems associated with the occurrence, or risk of occurrence, of a genetic disease or birth defect within a family. The multifaceted goals of this interaction include helping individuals and families to:

- Comprehend the medical facts including the diagnosis, the probable course of a disorder, and the available management
- Appreciate the way heredity contributes to the disorder, and the risk of recurrence
- Understand the options of dealing with the risk of recurrence (such as options for prenatal testing)
- Choose the course of action that seems most appropriate in view of the client's perceptions of risk, religion, life beliefs, and family goals
- Make the best possible adjustment to the disorder or the course of action the family has chosen

Genetic counseling can help make the difference in the adjustment of a person and family to a genetic diagnosis. As noted by Robert Louis Stevenson, "Life is not a matter of holding good cards, but of playing a poor hand well."

WHAT TO EXPECT FROM A GENETICS CONSULTATION

Clinical genetics professionals are typically physicians certified by the American Board of Medical Genetics and master's-level trained genetic counselors certified by the American Board of Genetic Counseling. Often a genetic evaluation includes members from a team of core specialists that may include medical geneticists, genetic counselors, nurses and nurse practioners, nutritionists, social workers, mental health professionals, and pastoral counselors.

A first visit for genetic counseling or a clinical genetic evaluation generally lasts 1 to 2 hours. A written summary of the appointment is often provided to the patient (and family if requested). At a minimum a genetic evaluation includes (adapted from Marymee et al., 1998):

- Obtaining and reviewing a family pedigree (usually a minimum of three generations). For complicated diagnoses, pedigrees may be obtained in advance on the phone.
- Obtaining and reviewing available medical records (and sometimes photographs) on the individual and extended family.
- Obtaining and reviewing a medical history (and developmental history as appropriate).
- Arranging for a physical examination of the patient and other family members (if indicated).

- Discussing options for available genetic testing or diagnostic procedures (including discussion of test sensitivity and specificity), and arranging for testing (as appropriate).
- Establishing a diagnosis or potential diagnosis.
- Reviewing of the inheritance pattern(s) and natural history of the condition, disease monitoring and management, any preventive measures, and reproductive options.
- Discussing of prenatal testing options.
- Assessing personal, social, religious, and ethnocultural issues including their relationship to the patient's feelings about genetic and prenatal testing and the consequences of such testing.
- Assessing possible ethical concerns such as confidentiality, disparate paternity, insurability, discrimination, employment issues, feelings about prenatal diagnosis, and presymptomatic testing of a minor individual.
- Referring to community resources.
- Referring to appropriate medical specialties, as needed.
- Supporting patient decisions in the context of individual values, beliefs, and goals.
- Arranging for genetic counseling and/or additional tests/evaluations on other family members, as needed.

Because of the potentially profound impact that a genetic diagnosis may have on the life of the individual being evaluated, results are usually given in person. A follow-up visit or phone call to discuss the patient and family's reaction to the results is often advisable. If the results are the opposite of what the person (or family) anticipated they would be, there may be trouble adjusting to this new self-identity or state of being. Kessler (1988) describes this phenomenon as "preselection." Such individuals may regret past life choices that they might have made differently had they had prior knowledge of their genetic status.

Even "good news" can have a "negative" impact. The person may feel an unwelcome burden to take care of his or her affected relatives (both physically and financially). A healthy sibling may have a profound sense of "survivor guilt," wondering why he or she has "escaped" the disease whereas his or her siblings have been less fortunate. The "survivor" may feel on the outskirts of the "family team" despite knowing it is irrational to desire ill health.

LOCATING A GENETICS PROFESSIONAL

The National Society of Genetic Counselors (NSGC) is the leading voice, authority, and advocate for the genetic counseling profession. The NSGC has an on-line resource directory of master's-level trained genetic services providers in the United States and abroad. Providers can be located by city and state, as well as by subspecialty (such as prenatal diagnosis, neurogenetics, and cancer genetics). The URL is http://www.nsgc.org/resource_link.html. For more information contact: NSGC, 233 Canterbury Drive, Wallingford PA 19086-6617, Voice-mail (610)-872-7608, FAX (610) 872-1192, and E-mail nsgc@aol.com.

An up-to-date listing of genetics professionals in the United States and abroad can be accessed through the following Web sites (also refer to the Internet resources in Appendix A.5: The Genetics Library):

Helix: Genetic Testing Resource   http://www.genetests.org/

GeneClinics   http://www.geneclinics.org

Information for Genetics Professionals   http://www.kumc.edu/gec/geneinfo/html

Online Resource Center   http://www.pitt.edu/~edugene/resource/

These sites also have information about the 10 regional genetics networks in the United States, that are supported by the Maternal and Child Health Bureau, Health Resources and Services Administration, U.S. Department of Health and Human Services. These networks are a source of information on local resources in a variety of areas in human genetics. Because the regional genetics network offices are grant funded, the contact information is subject to change. There are hypertext links to all of the regional genetics networks at the Web sites listed above.

Information about the professional genetics societies including the American Society of Human Genetics, the American College of Medical Genetics, and the European Society of Human Genetics can be found on the World of Genetics Societies Homepage, <http://www.faseb.org/genetics/>. Information about the International Society of Nurses in Genetics is available at: ISONG, 7 Haskins Road, Hanover, NH 03755, telephone: 603-643-3028.

REFERENCES

Ad Hoc Committee on Genetic Counseling (1975). Report to the American Society of Human Genetics. Am J Hum Genet 27:240–242.

Costello AJ (1988). The psychosocial impact of genetic disease. In University of Colorado Health Sciences Center, *Genetics Applications: A Health Perspective.* Lawrence, KS: Learner Managed Designs, pp. 149–165.

Jonsen AR, Durfy SJ, Burke W, Motulsky AG (1996). The advent of the "unpatients." Nat Med 2(6):622–624.

Kessler S (1988). Invited essay on the psychological aspects of genetic counseling. V. Preselection: A family coping strategy in Huntington disease. Am J Med Genet 31:617–621.

Marymee K, Dolan CR, Pagon RA, Bennett RL, Coe S, Fisher N (1998). Development of the critical elements of genetic evaluation and genetic counseling for genetic professionals and perinatologists in Washington State. J Genet Couns 6:133–165.

Olshansky S (1962). Chronic sorrow: a response to having a mentally retarded child. Social Casework 43:190–193.

Plumridge D, Bennett R, Dinno N, Branson C (1993). *The Student With a Genetic Disorder: Educational Implications for Special Education Teachers and For Physical Therapists, Occupational Therapists, and Speech Pathologists.* Springfield: Charles C Thomas.

Pollen DA (1993). *Hannah's Heirs.* New York: Oxford University Press, pp. 33, 35.

Schild S, Black RB (1984). *Social Work and Genetics: A Guide For Practice.* New York: The Hawthorth Press.

10

Pedigree Predicaments

So tangled is the web we weave when once we practice to perceive.
—*Michael Bérubé (1997)*

THE "TRUTH"

A pedigree is unique from other components of a medical record because it contains personal information about extended family members that may or may not be absolutely factual. Although most pedigrees are probably reasonable representations of the "truth," each pedigree will vary slightly depending on the patient's recall of family data. For example, if my family physician were to record my medical-family history and compare it to a pedigree taken by my first cousin's primary care provider, the framework of the two pedigrees would be similar, but the family embellishments would undoubtedly vary. I certainly am more of an authority on my own health and the health and ages of my immediate family than I am on the health of my cousin's siblings and parents, and vice versa.

A health professional who provides care for multiple members in the same family may encounter a dilemma in how to record a pedigree when the "family facts" vary from one family member to another. Our clinic is a geographic hub for the diagnosis and care of many individuals with rare inherited disorders, thus we often provide services to persons from multiple branches of the same family. Although it is rewarding to follow the generations of an extended family over several years, I also find myself in some awkward situations. On several occasions during the patient interview I discover that I know more about the family of the patient sitting in the chair across from me than he or she does. I never know whether to record the pedigree as absolutely reported to me by the patient, or to correct the inaccuracies on the pedigree based on information received from family members seen at prior visits. The balance between protecting patient confidentiality and privacy, weighed against accuracy of patient information, is delicate.

As health professionals we all wear the blinders of our specialty; we naturally seek responses from a patient in relation to our field of expertise. This will influence the scope of the information recorded on a pedigree. I recall Mr. and Mrs. C, a couple referred to our genetics clinic by a respected local pediatric geneticist who had diagnosed the couple's first child, Anthony, with a lethal unbalanced chromosome rearrangement shortly before Anthony died in the newborn intensive care unit. We planned to continue the evaluation of the family by obtaining a chromosome study on each parent to determine if one of them carried a balanced chromosome rearrangement, and to proceed with further family studies if a chromosomal rearrangement was identified. When I greeted the couple in the lobby to escort them to my office, I was puzzled when one of our patients with Huntington disease rose to join them—she was Mr. C's mother! When the initial pedigree had been taken, the fact that Mr. C had Huntington disease in his family was neither solicited by the geneticist nor volunteered by Mr. and Mrs. C. The chromosome studies found that Mrs. C, two of her siblings, and her father carried a rare balanced reciprocal translocation. We were able to discuss the implications of the inheritance of both Huntington disease and the chromosome translocation for future pregnancies. A year later, Mrs. C phoned me with the nervous news that she was six weeks along in her pregnancy. She was interested in scheduling an appointment to discuss prenatal testing. After scheduling the appointment, Mrs. C said, " I have one more question, is hemophilia genetic?" When I asked her why she was asking she replied, "Oh, because two of my brothers and my mother's brother have hemophilia. I'm not really worried about it, I was just curious." How did two genetic professionals miss this classic X-linked genetic disease in the family history? The C's probably did not think that the information was important at the time of their visit and the genetic specialists (including me) were guilty of tunnel vision.

The choice of information that is recorded on a pedigree is biased by the cultural and scientific belief systems of the recorder. For example, whether or not I document information on a pedigree about cigarette smoking in family members depends on the family's disease. Given the causal association with tobacco usage and disease, I certainly would make pedigree notations regarding family members' usage of tobacco if my client was interested in a hereditary cancer risk assessment (Trizna and Schantz, 1998), or if he or she were inquiring about familial risks associated with cleft lip and palate (Shaw et al., 1996). I might not record information about the tobacco habits of family members at risk for Huntington disease because my scientific belief system does not register an association with the development of Huntington disease and the use of tobacco products. If a client informs me that a relative has attention deficit disorder, I would record this information on the pedigree if fragile X were a consideration in the family, but I might not if the concern was cystic fibrosis.

Historically pedigrees have been considered as a way of recording absolute truths. At the turn of the 20th century, the Eugenic Record Office (ERO) at Cold Spring Harbor was filled with serious and responsible scientists concerned about the civic duties of science and its application to human problems. Pedigrees were a part of this movement because they could demonstrate, as eugenicist Karl Pearson put it, "the raw facts of heredity, free of all more or less contentious interpretations" (Mazumdar, 1992). The early pioneers of pedigrees distributed standardized forms on "How to Make A Eugenical Family History" to the general public to encourage people to "register their family network." Families and their physicians were charged to describe both the good qualities and defects of family members with "care, accuracy, and frankness." Some of the objective traits to be marked were meanness, feeblemindedness, epilepsy, and alcoholism (Mazumdar, 1992). A quantitative measure of "meanness" is a challenge even in modern times! In hindsight we look at these historical pedigrees, taken by well meaning geneticists intending to better the world with science, and we shudder at the realization that herein lie the tarnished roots of the Nazi eugenic pogroms of the 1930s and 1940s.

My own style of recording pedigrees has evolved over time in synchrony with changes in my scientific knowledge. Ten years ago, if I were taking a family history from a woman whose mother died of breast cancer at age 42 years, I probably would have commented to her, "That must have been a difficult time for you." I may have asked, "Is there any other cancer in the family?" Even if the consultand replied "Yes," I probably would not have explored the family history any further, beyond saying, "You should be diligent with your breast self-exams, and follow the national screening guidelines for the early detection of breast and other cancers." Today, given the availability of genetic testing for some inherited cancer susceptibilities, I would ask a whole cascade of medical-family history questions (as outlined in Chapter 5), to try to identify patterns of a familial cancer syndrome. Ten years ago, when I saw a client with a family history of Huntington disease, I fanatically recorded the names and medical records of everyone in the family. At that time, blood had to be obtained from multiple family members in more than one generation because presymptomatic testing required DNA linkage analysis. I recorded the state they lived in because I might need a blood sample from those family members. Now, with direct DNA testing for Huntington disease, I am less focused on the names of the extended family, and I am more focused on satisfying that the family pedigree appears autosomal dominant and that an affected family member has had a positive DNA test. Just as family dynamics change, so does our focus in genetics.

THE RESEARCHER AND FAMILY STUDIES

Because specialists in all medical disciplines care for individuals with genetic disorders, any health professional may someday be involved with a person participating in a genetic research study. Research studies in which a subject has a genetic disorder (or potentially inherited condition) are different from the study of an individual for a nongenetic indication. Table 10.1 compares the traditional model of individual subject research to that of a family studies model (Frankel and Teich, 1993). Areas of subject recruitment, voluntary consent, and subject withdrawal must be carefully considered when research involves individuals and families with inherited disorders. Genetic research of minor children should be approached with particular caution. Because the study results may affect multiple family members, a discussion of

TABLE 10.1   Unique Issues in Family Studies

Traditional Research Model

1. Subject has no ties to other research participants
2. Information learned from the research affects only the subject
3. Subject consents to be studied as an individual
4. Subject recruitment is entirely voluntary and is usually based on specific "medical" features under study
5. Subject can withdraw from study at any time for any reason

Family Studies Model

1. Subject has ties to other research participants because of shared genetic heritage
2. Information learned from research affects the family, and what researchers learn about the family affects what the subject knows about self
3. Other family members become part of study without their consent because they are members of a family under study
4. Subject recruitment may not be entirely voluntary because other family member(s) may "benefit" if family members participate; therefore, subject may feel "coercion" to participate from the other family member(s) already participating in study
5. Although subject can withdraw from study (i.e., by requesting destruction of subject's blood/tissue sample), how can one withdraw/destroy family history information? Does that mean if one person withdraws, the whole family must withdraw from the study?

Source: Adapted from Frankel and Teich, 1993.

if, how, and to whom results will be given must be a critical component of the informed consent process.

PEDIGREES AND PUBLICATIONS

It is common to publish a pedigree as part of a case study or genetic research. The pedigree can be a powerful and succinct presentation of scientific data. Caution must be used to protect privacy and confidentiality of family members in the decision to publish a pedigree.

Two groups have addressed the complex issues of privacy and confidentiality in the publication of pedigrees. In a 1993 guidebook, The National Institute of Health's Office for Protection from Research Risks (OPRR) addresses the issues of publication of pedigrees by stating, "Where a risk of identification exists, participants must consent, in writing, to the release of personal information." Furthermore, Institutional Review Boards (IRB's) should address the following questions:

1. Is the pedigree essential to the publication?
2. Can identifying data be omitted?
3. If an identifying pedigree is to be published, have subjects given consent for publication?

Guidelines by the International Committee of Medical Journal Editors (ICMJE) released in 1995 state:

> Patients have rights to privacy that should not be infringed without informed consent. Identifying information should not be published in written descriptions, photographs, or pedigrees unless the information is essential for scientific purposes and the patient (or parent or guardian) gives written informed consent for publication. Informed consent for this purpose requires that the patient be shown the manuscript to be published. Identifying details should be omitted if they are not essential, but patient data should never be altered or falsified in an attempt to attain anonymity. Complete anonymity is difficult to achieve, and informed consent should be obtained if there is any doubt. For example, masking of the eye region in photographs of patients is inadequate protection of anonymity. The requirement of informed consent should be included in the journal's instructions for authors. When informed consent has been obtained it should be indicated in the published article.

The practice of masking or altering pedigrees to protect privacy and confidentiality is controversial. Botkin and colleagues define "masking" as using symbols in a way that is obvious to the reader that information is being withheld; such as choosing diamonds to "mask" the sex of individuals or giving approximate instead of absolute ages. The purpose of masking could be compared to using black bands across the eyes to "disguise" a patient in a published photograph. In contrast, "alteration" is used in reference to changing symbols or the framework of a pedigree in ways that may not be evident to the reader, for example, altering the birth order, changing gender, or not including all members of a sibship (Botkin et al., 1998).

One of the earliest examples of an altered pedigree is a pedigree published by the Eugenics Education Society showing the inheritance of brilliance and scientific ability in Darwin's own family (Fig. 10.1). The pedigree is striking for its holandric (Y-linked) inheritance of ability in that only the male relatives are gifted. If one compares this pedigree to Figure 3.11 you will note the pedigree is biased by the absence of some contributory family facts including mental retardation in Darwin's youngest son and in his mother's sister. Other missing information is alcoholism in multiple family members, and hereditary deafness in the Wedgwood family (Bowlby, 1992; Resta, 1995). The pedigree data may have been modified by Darwin's son Leonard (who was president of the Eugenic Education Society) to bolster the theory of the hereditary nature of his own family's genius (Robert Resta, personal communication).

A well-known example of a pedigree that was masked and altered in a nationally recognized journal was a pedigree diagram published in 1987 by Dr. Nancy Wexler and colleagues of a couple that each had Huntington disease. Their 14 children were represented as diamonds on the pedigree as a way of showing that four of the 14 siblings were homozygous for the HD allele. The pedigree was published in this manner to protect the privacy of these homozygous individuals because 100% of their children are at risk to develop Huntington disease. Until the publication of this pedigree, it was unknown whether or not individuals who are homozygous for the HD alleles would be more severely affected than a heterozygous individual (the answer

CHART SHOWING THE
INHERITANCE OF ABILITY

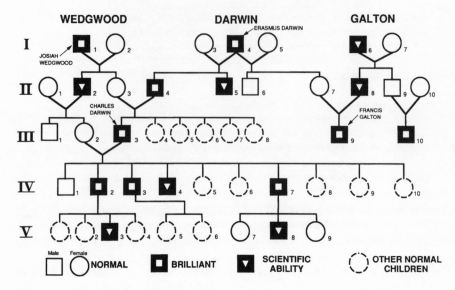

Figure 10.1 *A pedigree of the Wedgwood–Darwin–Galton family. Generation and individual numbers and names have been added to the original pedigree for ease in identification. Courtesy of Robert Resta, reprinted from P Mazumdar (1992) with permission from Routledge, Chapman and Hall, Inc.*

was no). By publishing this altered pedigree to protect family confidentiality, was the integrity of the scientific information compromised? We may never know.

By altering or masking pedigrees, valuable information may be lost. For example, researchers who are studying the phenomenon of anticipation in a specific disease often review published pedigrees to determine whether or not there is a trend for earlier ages of disease onset and more severe disease in successive generations. To recognize diseases with imprinting or mitochondrial inheritance, it is critical to record the sex of the transmitting parent. If the ages and sexes of individuals on the pedigree are altered, important patterns in disease expression may be missed or incorrectly interpreted.

One could argue that the practice of masking and altering pedigrees is "fudging" the data and is no more acceptable than if an investigator modifies aberrant research data to fit a hypothesis. A survey of investigators who published pedigrees in respectable scientific journals reports that 19% of 177 respondents have published an altered pedigree and 45% of these individuals did not disclose their alterations to the journal editor (Botkin et al., 1998).

All published pedigrees are "truncated;" an investigator must use discretion in how many generations in a pedigree are necessary to prove or illustrate the hypothesis. For example, a pedigree demonstrating familial Alzheimer disease might not include the grandchildren of affected individuals since they are not of an age to show symptoms. Likewise, a published pedigree will probably extend back only to the parents in the first affected generation even if more information is known about prior generations. If full genealogical charts were published, the pedigrees would be cluttered and fill costly journal space.

Who distinguishes which information is trivial to record on a pedigree? For example, information such as miscarriages or stillbirths may seem irrelevant to the disease under study, yet a certain genotype may be lethal at the embryonic stage. There is a fuzzy line between the protection of identifying information and the reporting of "pure" data.

One should assume that any pedigree is potentially identifiable. Also, because the lay public has easy access to medical literature through the Internet and through communication with patient disease advocacy groups, one must assume that any patient or family members may see their published pedigree. Here are some points to consider if you are in the position to publish a pedigree, if you are reviewing an article for publication in a journal, or if you are part of your institution's human subjects review board:

- Did family members give consent for the publication of a pedigree? If so, were they shown a copy of the pedigree that will be published?
- Does the pedigree contain sensitive information that is unknown to the subject (for example, presymptomatic testing information or information on minor children)?
- Does the pedigree add to the understanding of the publication? Does it contain the necessary information needed to support or refute the hypothesis?
- Could family members find out information from the pedigree that they do not already know? For example, does the pedigree disclose results of presymptomatic testing that the person has not been given, or might other family members find out information about a risk to themselves that they were not aware of?
- And, perhaps the most telling question—if this were your family pedigree, would you be upset by disclosure of the information?

SUMMARY

Medical-family histories are a critical component of clinical medicine and research. Recording this information in the form of a pedigree is a shorthand method of tracking key elements (such as age, health status, and environmental exposures) in multiple family members in several generations. Because the identification of a genetic disorder in a family can be perceived as a stigma by the family and "society," there are unique ethical issues to consider in the delivery of clinical services, the provision of informed consent for participation in research studies, and the publication of pedigrees.

The medical-family history information that is elicited from a patient and then recorded on a pedigree is prejudiced by the cultural and scientific belief systems of both the patient and the health care provider. Is documenting information on a pedigree, such as misattributed paternity, depression, sexual orientation, abortions, drug and alcohol abuse, behavioral problems, and criminal behavior, a record of medical facts or social information? Our biases may not be easily recognized, as Resta (1995) notes:

> ... In genetics, as in all scientific pursuits, the construction and interpretation of a pedigree can be influenced by the political and social beliefs of all-too-human geneticists. Those beliefs may be so ingrained that we mistake them for biological laws. It is, I suspect, beyond our ability to know which of our personal biases we are disguising as scientific truths. The whisper and hints of our biases may be heard only by future generations. . . .

REFERENCES

Botkin JR, McMahon WM, Smith KR, Nash JE (1998). Privacy and confidentiality in the publication of pedigrees: a survey of investigators and biomedical journals. JAMA 279:1808–1812.

Bowlby, John (1992). Charles Darwin: A New Life. New York, London: W. W. Norton and Company.

Frankel MS, Teich, Art (1993). Ethical and Legal Issues in Pedigree Research. Washington, DC: American Association for the Advancement of Science.

International Committee of Medical Journal Editors (1995). Protection of patient's rights to privacy. BMJ 311:1272.

Mazumdar PMH (1992). *Eugenics, Human Genetics and Human Failings.* London, New York: Routledge.

Office for Protection from Research Risks (1993). Protecting Human Research Subjects: Institutional Review Board Guidebook. U.S. Government Printing Office, Washington, DC. 5-42—5-56.

Resta R (1995). Whispered hints. Am J Med Genet 59:131–133

Shaw GM, Wasserman CR, Lammer EJ, et al., (1996). Orofacial clefts, parental cigarette smoking, and transforming growth factor-alpha gene variants. Am J Hum Genet 58:551–561.

Trizna Z, Schantz S (1998). Tobacco-related cancers of the respiratory and upper digestive tract. In: Foulkes WD, Hodgson SV (eds), *Inherited Susceptibility to Cancer: Clinical, Predictive and Ethical Perspectives.* Cambridge: Cambridge University Press.

Wexler NS, Young AB, Tanz RE, et al. (1987). Homozygotes for Huntington's disease. Nature 326:194–197.

Glossary

acanthocytosis   The presence in the blood of distorted red cells with a "thorny" appearance

age of onset   Age at which the effects of a genetic disorder become evident

allele   Alternative forms of the gene occupying a specific site on a chromosome

allelic heterogeneity   Multiple gene mutations at the same locus that are each capable of producing an aberrant phenotype

amino acids   The major building blocks of polypeptides. Each of the 20 amino acids is encoded by one or more mRNA codons

amniocentesis   Removal, through a needle inserted through the abdomen and uterus, of a small amount of the amniotic fluid, which is analyzed for fetal testing

amniotic bands   Strands of tissue, thought to be from the rupture of the amnion (the sac around the fetus), leading to disruption of fetal development resulting in asymmetric congenital abnormalities (such as amputated digits, facial clefting)

anal atresia   (imperforate anus) Congenital absence of an anal opening

anencephaly   Failure of the anterior neural tube to close, leading to complete or partial absence of the cranial vault (forebrain, overlying meninges, skull, and skin); a neural tube defect

aneuploidy   Cells that contain a variant of the normal diploid number of 46 chromosomes (either extra or missing chromosomes) Triploidy with 69 chromosomes is a polyploidy

aniridia   Absence of the iris of the eye

anophthalmos   Congenital absence of the eyes or the presence of a vestigial eye

anosmia   Absence of smell

anotia   Congenital absence of the pinna (external ears)

anticipation   The observation in a pedigree of a disease occurring at earlier ages or with increased severity in successive generations. In many instances this is attributed to an unstable trinucleotide repeat

arachnodactyly   Long thin fingers or toes

artificial insemination   See *therapeutic insemination*

arthrogryposis Congenital joint contractures

Ashkenazi Jews whose ancestors were from Central and Eastern Europe

assortative mating A term used by geneticists to explain that humans do not choose their mating partners randomly

asymptomatic carrier A person who carries a gene alteration but will not develop the disease

ataxia Poor coordination of movement with a wide-based, unsteady gait often associated with poor coordination of the limbs and speech

atresia Congenital absence or closure of a normal body orifice or tubular organ (e.g., anal atresia, esophageal atresia)

autosome The 22 pairs of chromosomes excluding the sex chromosomes (X and Y)

azoospermia The absence of sperm in the seminal fluid; may be due to a blockage or an impairment of sperm production

benign A tumor that does not invade surrounding tissue

bifid uvula A cleft in the uvula; a minor manifestation of cleft palate. The *uvula* is the small, conical, fleshy mass of tissue suspended from the center of the soft palate above the back of the tongue

brachydactyly Abnormal shortness of the fingers and/or toes

branchial cysts or fistulas Vestiges of the embryonic branchial grooves. Found in the lower third of the neck, and may be bilateral. They are associated with hearing loss, specifically with the branchio-oto-renal (BOR) syndrome

brushfield spots Speckled, mottled, or marbled rings about two-thirds of the distance to the periphery of the iris

café au lait spots Area of brown skin pigmentation with irregular borders

canthus Inner or outer edge of the eye (as in inner canthus or outer canthus)

carrier An individual who has one copy of a disease causing gene but does not express the disease. An *asymptomatic carrier* is someone who is not expected to develop the disease (e.g., a woman who carries a fragile X mutation). A *presymptomatic carrier* is someone who is expected to develop the disease sometime in his or her lifetime (e.g., Huntington disease)

chorionic villus sampling (CVS) A technique for obtaining tissue from the developing placenta (the chorionic villi) for the purpose of prenatal testing usually performed at 10–12 weeks gestation

choroid The dark brown vascular coat of the eye between the sclera (white of the eye) and the retina (the light sensitive membrane of the inner eyeball)

clinical heterogeneity The existence of clinically different phenotypes from mutations in the same gene

clinodactyly An incurving finger

coarctation of the aorta Narrowing of either a short or long segment of the aorta near the area of the ductus arteriosus

codominance The expression of both alleles in a heterozygous individual

codon A group of three mRNA bases, each of which specifies an amino acid when translated

coloboma A fissure (cleft or groove) especially of the eye (may involve the iris, retina, lid, etc.) which can be congenital or traumatic in origin. An iris coloboma has a "keyhole" appearance

conductive hearing loss   Hearing loss caused by a physical problem of the external and/or middle ear

congenital   A characteristic that is present at birth (not necessarily inherited)

consanguinity   In medical genetics, used to refer to any union between biological relatives (i.e., first cousins). The term *incest* is usually reserved for sexual unions between couples who are related as first degree relatives (e.g., father-daughter, brother-sister)

consultand   The individual seeking genetic services. The consultand may or may not be affected

contiguous gene syndrome   A disease associated with a microscopic deletion or duplication involving several consecutive genes located on a chromosome arm. See *microdeletion syndrome*

craniosynostosis   An abnormally shaped head due to premature fusion of the cranial bones

cubitis valgus   Increased carrying angle at the elbow

cystic hygroma(s)   Congenital cyst(s) of the lymphatic system most commonly found within the soft tissues of the neck

deformation   An abnormal shape or position of a part of the body caused by in utero mechanical forces

deletion   A missing sequence of DNA or part of a chromosome

dementia   A general description for mental deterioration

diaphragmatic hernia   Some portion of the abdominal contents protrude through the diaphragm into the chest cavity

diploid   Cells possessing pairs of chromosomes (two of each type)

disruption   The result of interference with an originally normal development process resulting in a birth defect

double-outlet right ventricle   Classification of a group of congenital heart defects in which both great arteries arise from the morphological right ventricle

DSM IV Classification   Abbreviation for *Diagnostic and Statistical Manual of Mental Disorders,* 4th Edition; a book containing diagnostic criteria for mental disorders

duodenal atresia   The absence, blocking, or narrowing of a portion of the duodenum (small bowel)

dynamic mutation   A gene mutation that is unstable when transmitted from parent to child. The term is usually used in reference to trinucleotide repeat disorders

dysarthria   Slurred speech

dysmorphic   A collection of unusual external features (usually seen in the head, hands, and face), which may be indicative of more serious internal problems

dysostosis multiplex   Defective ossification leading to a pattern of skeletal abnormalities including a large skull with a deep, elongated, J-shaped sella, oar-like ribs, deformed, hooked-shaped lower thoracic and upper lumbar vertebrae, pelvic dysplasia, shortened tubular bones with expanded diaphyses, and dysplastic epiphyses. A common characteristic of the mucopolysaccharide storage diseases.

dystonia Disordered muscle tone or tension

dystopia canthorum Short palpebral fissures with displacement of inner canthi giving impression of hypertelorism

Ebstein anomaly Displacement of the septal and posterior leaflets of the tricuspid valve toward the apex of the right ventricle

ectopia cordis The heart is totally (or partially) outside of the chest

ectopia lentis Dislocated lens(es) of the eye(s)

ectopic pregnancy An embryo that grows outside of the uterus, usually in a fallopian tube

empirical risk The probability that a trait will recur based upon its observed incidence in a particular population

encephalocele A type of neural tube defect in which brain tissue protrudes through a defect in the skull

encephalopathy A degenerative disease of the brain

endocardial cushion defect Term used to describe a spectrum of heart defects involving an atrial–septal defect (ASD) associated with ventricular septal defects (VSD) and abnormalities of the atrioventricular (AV) valves

epicanthal folds Congenital vertical fold of skin medial to the eye and lateral to the nose, sometimes covering the inner canthus

esophageal atresia A blind-ending esophageal pouch often associated with a traecheoesophageal fistula (TEF)

etiology Cause

expressivity The degree to which a heritable trait is expressed in an individual. The clinical severity of the trait(s)

exencephaly A problem with closure of the neural tube leading to the brain lying outside of the skull

exon Portion of genes that encode amino acids that are retained after the primary mRNA transcript is spliced

familial The occurrence of a trait in more than one family member at a greater frequency than expected by chance alone; not synonymous with hereditary

fibroids Noncancerous tumor composed mainly of fibrous or fully developed connective tissue

first degree relatives An individual's children, full brothers, full sisters, and parents

gamete An egg or a sperm

gastroschisis The intestine is entirely outside of the body through a defect in the umbilical wall

genome The entire sequence of an organism's DNA

genotype The genetic constitution of an individual as applied to a single locus or all the loci collectively

gestational carrier (surrogate) A woman who carries a fetus for a couple in her uterus with the intention of legally giving up the child to the couple at birth. She may also provide the oocytes

gonadal agenesis   Absent or rudimentary testis/testes, or ovary/ovaries

gonads   Sites of sperm and egg cell production (testes and ovaries, respectively)

gynecomastia   Excessive development of breast tissue in a male

hamartoma   A benign tumorlike nodule composed of an overgrowth of mature cells and tissues that normally occur in the affected body part or organ

hematuria   Blood in the urine

hemizygous   Possessing only one of a pair of genes that influence the determination of a particular trait. A *hemizygote* is a person who is hemizygous for a particular gene

hereditary   Traits under genetic control that may be transmitted to the next generation

hepatosplenomegaly   Enlarged liver and spleen

heterochromia   Different colored irises (i.e., one brown eye and one blue eye)

heterogeneity   The occurrence of the same or similar phenotypes from different genetic mechanisms

heterozygote   (heterozygous) An individual (or genotype) with two different alleles at a given locus

hirsute   Excessive body hair

historian   The person providing medical-family history information to the clinician

holoprosencephaly   A term used to describe the spectrum of anomalies resulting in abnormal cleavage of the embryonic forebrain and midline facial anomalies. Three subtypes are seen: alobar, lobar, and semilobar

homozygote   (homozygous) An individual (or genotype) with identical alleles at a given locus

hydrocephalus   Abnormal accumulation of cerebrospinal fluid within the cranial vault resulting in an enlarged head, prominent forehead, and usually mental deterioration and seizures

hypertelorism   An increased distance between two organs or parts, commonly used to refer to ocular hypertelorism (increased interpupillary distance)

hyperthermia   Abnormally high body temperature

hypoglycemia   Low level of blood sugar

hypogonadism   Small testes

hypoplasia   Incomplete development of an organ so that it fails to reach typical adult size

hypoplastic left-heart syndrome (HLHS)   Hypoplasia of the left ventricle associated with atresia or severe stenosis of the aortic arch and mitral valves with hypoplasia of the aortic arch

hypospadias   The opening of the penis is not at the tip of the penile shaft

hypotelorism   Decreased distance between two organs or body parts, commonly used to refer to ocular hypotelorism (decreased interpupillary distance)

hypotonia/hypotonic   Low muscle tone (floppy)

ICSI (intracytoplasmic sperm injection)   A procedure of therapeutic insemination where a single sperm is directly inserted into an individual egg

idiopathic   Of spontaneous origin

imprinting   The process by which genetic material is expressed differently when inherited from the father than when inherited from the mother

inborn error of metabolism   An inherited biochemical disorder resulting from a malfunctioning or absent enzyme in a metabolic pathway

incidence   An expression of the rate or frequency at which a certain event (or disease) occurs

index case   The first affected person to be studied in the family

individual's line   The vertical line in a pedigree extending up from an individual's symbol to connect to a *sibship line*. If an individual has no siblings, the individual's line connects directly to the horizontal relationship line. In this case the vertical *line of descent* and the individual's line are the same. Multiple births have a single individual's line that forks for each individual

iniencephaly   Extremely short cervical spine with missing vertebrae and extension of the fetal head in association with neural tube defects (e.g. anencephaly, meningomyelocele)

intron   The noncoding DNA sequence found between two exons. Introns are transcribed into primary mRNA but spliced out in the formation of the mature mRNA transcript

in utero   Within the uterus

inversion   A chromosome alteration in which a segment has been reversed because of breakage, 180° rotation, and reunion

ischemia   Deficiency of blood supply to a part of the body due to obstruction or constriction of a blood vessel

karyotype   The standardized arrangement of chromosome pairs in a single cell by number

key   Used in medical pedigrees to define unusual symbols and shading to assist with interpretation. Sometimes referred to as a *legend*

kindred   A family grouping

leiomyoma   A benign tumor (fibroid) usually found in the uterus

legend   See *key*

line of descent   The vertical line on a pedigree connecting the horizontal relationship line to the horizontal sibship line. If an individual does not have siblings, the line of descent and the individual's line is the same

lipoma   Fatty, benign tumor

locus   (plural, loci) The chromosomal location of a specific gene

macrocephaly   Unusually large head

macule   A flat, discolored spot on the skin

malformation   Defects in an organ, or part of an organ, resulting from an intrinsically abnormal development process

meconium   The dark-green intestinal waste in a full term fetus. Presence of meconium in the amniotic fluid is a sign of fetal distress

meningomyelocele   A common neural tube defect involving protrusion of the cord and its meninges through a defect in the vertebral canal

metastasis   The spread of malignant cells from one site in the body to another (the verb is metastasize)

methylation   The attachment of methyl group ($-CH_3$) to cytosine in DNA. Hyper-methylation of cytosine within or near a coding sequence is associated with a reduction in gene activity. Genes that are permanently active in all cells lack methyl groups

microcephaly   Unusually small head

microdeletion syndrome   A chromosome deletion that is too small to be visible under a microscope

micrognathia   Small, recessed jaw or chin

microphthalmos   Abnormally small eyes

microtia   Small, underdeveloped ear with a blind or absent external auditory canal

mitochondria   Small, spherical to rod-shaped organelles found in the cytoplasm (outside the nucleus) of cells. They are a major source of energy for the cell

monosomy   Missing one of a chromosome pair or partial chromosome pair in a normally diploid cell

mosaic   The existence of two or more genetically distinct cell lines in an individual

multifactorial   The interaction of many genes and the environment

mutation   A change in DNA sequence

myoclonus   Shock-like contractions of a muscle or muscle group

myopathy   Any disease of a muscle (e.g., cardiac myopathy)

myopia   Commonly referred to as nearsightedness

neonate   A newborn infant

neural tube   An embryonic structure that develops into the brain and spinal cord

neuropathy   A general term referring to functional or pathological changes in the peripheral nervous system

nevi   Moles

nitrogenous bases   Components of nucleic acids consisting of purines (adenine and guanine) and pyrimidines (cytosine, thymine, and uracil)

nondisjunction   Failure of chromosomes to separate properly in the process of mitosis or meiosis, resulting in cells or gametes with too few, or too many chromosomes

nonpaternity   The biological father is not as stated

nystagmus   Involuntary rapid movement of the eyeball (may be horizontal, vertical, mixed, or rotary)

obligate carrier   A person who carries a gene or chromosome alteration (known by pedigree analysis or genetic testing) who will not clinically manifest the disease

oligohydramnios   Decreased amniotic fluid. Anhydramnios is absence of amniotic fluid

oligozoospermia (oligospermia)   An abnormally low number of sperm in a semen sample

omphalocele   Protrusion of the intestines and/or other abdominal organs through a defect in the abdominal wall into a transparent sac

p   In cytogenetics, refers to the short arm of the chromosome (from the French petit)

palpebral fissures   Eye opening

paracentric inversion   A segment of a chromosome that is inverted but does not include the centromere (the site where the chromosome constricts)

pectus carinatum   Protrusion of the breastbone (sternum). Unflatteringly referred to as "pigeon breast"

pectus excavatum   Depression of the breastbone (sternum). Sometimes referred to as a "funnel chest"

pedigree   A diagrammatic representation of family relationships indicating health status

penetrance   The likelihood that a genetic condition is actually expressed in a population; usually phrased as a percentage of expression at a certain time (e.g., 60% penetrant at birth, 100% penetrant by age 40 years)

pericentric inversion   A segment of the chromosome that is inverted and includes the centromere (the site where the chromosome constricts)

periungual fibromas   Small wart-like tumors that develop around and under the finger and toenails; diagnostic of tuberous sclerosis

phakomatoses   A collection of disorders predisposing to hamartomas and other tumors involving the skins and/or eyes, nervous system, and one or more body systems. Derived from the Greek word "phakos" for mother-spot or birthmark

phenotype   The outward physical features of an individual

philtrum   Vertical groove in the midline of the upper lip, extending from underneath the nose to the top of the upper lip

polydactyly   Extra fingers or toes. *Postaxial polydactyly* means the extra finger is lateral to the fifth finger. *Preaxial polydactyly* means the extra digit is medial to the thumb

polygenic   A trait caused by the combined effects of multiple genes

polyhydramnios   Increased amount of amniotic fluid

premutation   An unstable allele that is not associated with disease

prenatal diagnosis   Testing to identify a disease or anomaly in a fetus or embryo

prevalence   The total number of cases of a disease in existence at a certain time in a designated area (e.g., the prevalence of Smith–Lemli–Opitz syndrome at birth among Caucasians in North America is 1/20,000)

proband   An affected family member coming to medical attention independent of other family members

prognathia   A protuding jaw

ptosis   Drooping of the upper eyelid

q   In cytogenetics, refers to the long arm of the chromosome

relationship line   The horizontal line on a pedigree joining "mating" partners. A break in this line indicates a divorce or separation in the union

renal agenesis   Absence of the kidney(s)

retina   A multilayer light-sensitive membrane lining the inner eyeball that sends visual signals to the brain through the optic nerve

ribosomes   Small particles in the cell cytoplasm serving as the sites of protein synthesis; they attach to the messenger RNA

sclerae   Whites of the eyes

scoliosis   Curvature of the spine; a lateral (sideways) deviation of the normally straight line of the spine

second degree relatives   An individual's aunts, uncles, grandparents, nieces and nephews, grandchildren, and half siblings

sex chromosomes   The X and Y chromosomes

sex-influenced gene expression   A gene whose expression is modified by the gender of the individual possessing the gene alteration (e.g., breast cancer)

sex-limited gene expression   A trait that is expressed only in one sex or the other

sex-linked   A gene that is located on the X or Y chromosome

sib   A brother or sister

siblings   An individual's brothers and sisters. Full siblings share the same mother and father

sibship line   The horizontal line used in a medical pedigree to connect individuals related as brothers and sisters (both full and half siblings). Each sibling is connected to the sibship line by a vertical *individual's line.* A vertical *line of descent* connects directly from the symbol for a parent (or from the horizontal *relationship line* between parents) to the sibship line

simian crease   A single palmar crease. (Typically individuals have a transverse double horizontal crease across each palm)

spasticity   Increased muscle tone

spina bifida   An early embryonic defect resulting in an opening anywhere along the spinal column

spontaneous pneumothorax   An accumulation of gas or air in the chest cavity that may lead to a collapsed lung

sporadic   The occurrence of a disease in a family with no apparent genetic transmission pattern

surrogate   See *gestational carrier*

syndactyly   Webbing or fusion of the fingers and/or toes

syndrome   A collection of characteristics that are recognized as a distinct clinical diagnosis

synophrys   Eyebrows (often bushy) that meet at the midline

telangiectasia   "Spider web" blood vessels, usually found on the skin and the whites of the eyes

teratogen   An environmental agent capable of causing malformations in the embryo

tetralogy of Fallot (TOF)   The combination of a ventricular septal defect (VSD) with pulmonary stenosis at the infundibular level (with or without associated valve stenosis), and right ventricular hypertrophy with an aorta that overrides the ventricular septal defect

therapeutic insemination   (TI) A means of conceiving a pregnancy whereby the semen is obtained from the male and placed into a woman's reproductive tract. This term is preferred over the commonly used term artificial insemination

third degree relatives   An individual's first cousins, great grandparents, half aunts and half uncles, great grandchildren, and great aunts and great uncles

tracheoesophageal fistula (TEF)   An abnormal passageway between the trachea and the esophagus

translocation   A chromosome rearrangement between two chromosomes

transposition of the great vessels   The aorta arises entirely from the right ventricle and the pulmonary artery from the left ventricle, resulting in complete separation of the circulations

trinucleotide repeat   A repeated sequence of three bases (e.g., CAG, CCG) that is expanded and unstable in some genetic disorders (triplet repeat disorders)

trisomy   An extra copy of all or part of a chromosome normally present in a diploid state

uniparental disomy   Both copies of a chromosome pair are inherited from the same parent instead of inheriting one copy of each chromosome pair from the mother and the father

URL   The address of a site on the Internet

variable expression   A trait in which the same genotype may produce phenotypes with different manifestations and severity

velopharyngeal insufficiency   Referring to the incompetence of the soft palate, indicative of a submucosal cleft. Often evidenced by a nasal speech tone

ventricular septal defect   Absence of part or all of the wall (septum) between the ventricles (lower chambers) of the heart

xanthoma   A yellow colored nodule, papule, or plaque in the skin due to lipid deposits

X-linked   Genes that are located on the X chromosome

Y-linked   Genes that are located on the Y chromosome

Handy Reference Tables of Pedigree Nomenclature

Some of these figures were previously published in Bennett et al., American Journal of Human Genetics, 56:745–52, 1995 and are republished with permission of the University of Chicago Press.

STANDARDIZED SYMBOLS AND NOMENCLATURE FOR HUMAN PEDIGREES
(Adapted from Bennett RL et. al., Am J Hum Genet, 56:7445, 1995)

Information to include in a pedigree

- Age/birth date, or year of birth
- Age at death (year if known)
- Cause of death
- Full sibs versus half sibs
- Relevant health information (e.g., height, weight)
- Age at diagnosis
- Affected/unaffected status (define shading of symbol in key/legend)
- Personally evaluated or medically documented (*)
- Testing status ("E" is used for evaluation on pedigree and defined in key/legend)
- Pregnancies with gestational age noted LMP or EDD - estimated date of delivery
- Pregnancy complications with gestational age noted (e.g., 6 wk, 34 wk), miscarriage (SAB), stillbirth (SB), pregnancy termination (TOP), ectopic (ECT)
- Infertility vs. no children by choice
- Ethnic background of each grandparent
- Use a "?" if family history is unknown
- Consanguinity (note degree of relationship if not implicit in pedigree
- Family names (if appropriate)
- Date pedigree taken
- Name of person who took pedigree and credentials (MD, RN, MSW, CGC)
- Key/legend

Pedigree Symbols

	Male	Female	Sex Unkown
Individual (assign gender by phenotype)	□ b. 1925	○ 30	◇ 4 mo
Clinically affected individual (define shading in key/legend)	■	●	◆
Affected individual (> one condition)	▨	◔	◈
Multiple individuals, number known	5	5	5
Multiple individuals, number unknown	n	n	n
Deceased individual	⊘ d. 35 y	⊘ d. 4 mo	⬨
Stillbirth (SB)	⊘ SB 28 wk	⊘ SB 30 wk	⬨ SB 34 wk
Pregnancy (P)	P LMP: 7/1/94	P 20 wk	P 16 wk
Spontaneous abortion (SAB), ectopic (ECT)	△ male	△ female	△ ECT
Affected SAB	▲ male	▲ female	▲ 16 wk
Termination of pregnancy (TOP)	⟋△ male	⟋△ female	⟋△ 12 wk
Affected TOP	▲ male	▲ female	▲ 12 wk
Consultand	↗□ b. 4/24/59	↗○ 35y	
Proband	P↗■	P↗●	

STANDARDIZED SYMBOLS AND NOMENCLATURE FOR HUMAN PEDIGREES
(Adapted from Bennett RL et al., Am J Hum Genet, 56:7445, 1995)

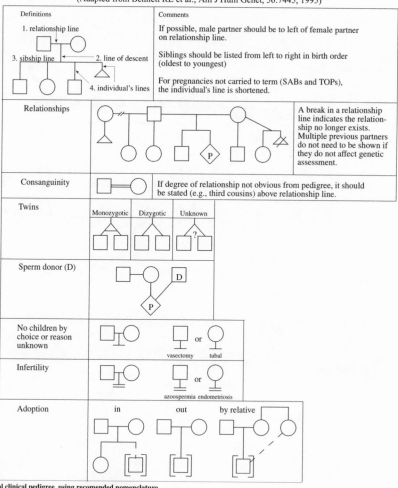

Hypothetical clinical pedigree, using recomended nomenclature

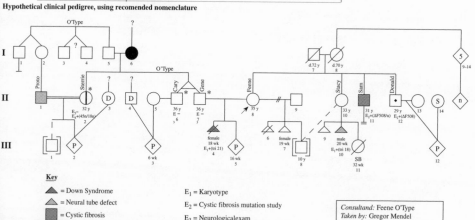

Key

▲ = Down Syndrome

△ = Neural tube defect

▨ = Cystic fibrosis

▦ = Red/green color blindness

● = Huntington disease (affected)

▯ = Huntington disease (presymptomatic)

⊡ = Cystic fibrosis asymptomatic carrier

E_1 = Karyotype

E_2 = Cystic fibrosis mutation study

E_3 = Neurologicalexam

E_4 = Huntington disease mutation study

* = Examined personally

S = Surrogate mother

D = Gamete donor

Consultand: Feene O'Type
Taken by: Gregor Mendel
Historians: Gene and Feene O'Type
Date of intake: April 1, 1998

Sample Clinical Pedigree Form

FAMILY PEDIGREE   Record #: _____   Medical Center Location: _____

Consultand: _____   Historian: _____   Recorder: _____   Date: ___

Diagnosis: _____   KEY: ☐ -

Ancestry: _____   Consanguinity? _____   ☐ -

Sample Genetic Screening Form for Familial Cancer Risk Assessment

This form can be completed by healthy individuals or persons with cancer to assist the health care provider in identifying individuals who might be at an increased risk to develop cancer or another primary tumor. For those individuals with a possible contributory history (see Chapter 5 and Tables 5.1 and 5.2) a personal interview and the recording of a pedigree can explore the family history further.

Familial Cancer Risk Assessment Form

Date _____

Patient # _____

Name _____ Birthdate _____ Phone _____

Street Address _____ City _____ State _____ Zip _____

Your answers to the following questions will help us evaluate you and your family's cancer risk. We are interested in <u>any</u> cancer in a blood relative (for example, breast, colon, lung, uterine, pancreatic, prostate, ovarian, skin cancer, leukemia or lymphoma). A **maternal relative** is on your mother's side of the family. A **paternal relative** is on your father's side of the family.

Have you or any of the following blood relatives ever had cancer?

Relative	Living?	Type(s) of cancer	Age when cancer(s) found
Yourself		_____	_____
Mother	yes no	_____	_____
Maternal grandmother	yes no	_____	_____
Maternal grandfather	yes no	_____	_____
Father	yes no	_____	_____
Paternal grandmother	yes no	_____	_____
Paternal grandfather	yes no	_____	_____

How many blood-related **sisters** do you have? _____
How many of them have ever had cancer? _____
For each blood-related sister who had cancer, list the type(s), and her age when the cancer was found. For a half sister, write *M* for maternal or *P* for paternal.

Sister	Half?	Living?	Type(s) of cancer	Age when cancer found
1	___	yes no	_____	_____
2	___	yes no	_____	_____
3	___	yes no	_____	_____

How many blood-related **brothers** do you have? _____
How many of them have ever had cancer? _____
For each blood-related brother who had cancer, list the type(s), and his age when the cancer was found.

Brother	Half?	Living?	Type(s) of cancer	Age when cancer found
1	___	yes no	_____	_____
2	___	yes no	_____	_____
3	___	yes no	_____	_____

Turn Page Over and Continue

Name _____   **Page 2**

How many blood-related **children** do you have? _____
How many of them ever had cancer? _____
For each of your blood-related children who had cancer, list the type(s), and how old
he or she was when the cancer was found.

child #	Living?	Type(s) of cancer	Age when cancer found
1	yes no	_____	_____
2	yes no	_____	_____
3	yes no	_____	_____

Do you have any **other blood relatives** who have had cancer?   Yes   No
For each of your other blood relatives who have had cancer, list how he or she is related to you (your maternal aunt, paternal uncle, maternal first cousin, etc.), the
type(s) of cancer, and how old he or she was when the cancer was found.

Relation	Living?	Type(s) of cancer	Age when cancer found
_____	yes no	_____	_____
_____	yes no	_____	_____
_____	yes no	_____	_____

Have ANY of your relatives had breast cancer in *both* breasts?   Yes   No
If yes, which relative(s)? _____

Have any of your relatives had polyps in the colon or rectum?   Yes   No
If yes, which relative(s)? _____

To what country do you trace your ancestors (for example, France, Germany, China,
African American, Mexico)?
Your Mother's Father _____ *Your Mother's Mother* _____
Your Father's Father _____ *Your Father's Mother* _____

Is your family of Jewish descent (circle one)?   Yes   No   Don't know

Would you be interested in scheduling a genetics consultation regarding your family's history of cancer?   Yes   No   Maybe

Do you have any additional concerns?

APPENDIX *A.4*

Sample Adoption Medical-Family History Form

MODEL MEDICAL-GENETIC HISTORY FORM FOR ADOPTIONS

This model medical-genetic family history form is intended for use in adoptions. It is assumed that each user of this model form will modify it to comply with local or state regulations.

In documenting medical-genetic histories, it is optimal if EACH birth parent is assisted in completing the questionnaires by a trained adoption professional who appreciates the importance of collecting this information, and has an awareness of the medical and genetic conditions contained in the form.

The form consists of the following segments:

- A *Cover Page,* that contains identifying information about the birth parents child welfare agency, and an agency file identification code. This page is filed with the agency designated in each state to retain such identifying information. The cover page is not intended to be shared with the child who is adopted, nor with the adopting family, unless the birth parents agree to waive their right to confidentiality.
- A one-page *Pregnancy Care Information Sheet* to be completed by the birth mother.
- A one-page *Delivery, Birth, and Medical Information Sheet* to be completed by the birth mother or the adoption professional.
- An eight page *Medical-Genetic Family History Questionnaire.* One copy of this form should be completed by EACH birth parent.

The development of this form was supported in part by the CORN Education Committee, Project #: NCJ-361011-03 and was revised with permission by Robin L. Bennett, M.S., April 1998.

Joan Burns, M.S., M.S.S.W.	Diane Plumridge, M.S.W.
Robin L. Bennett, M.S.	Cheryl Schroeder, Ed.D.
Barbara Bernhardt, M.S.	Kerry Silvey, M.A.
Kathleen Delp, M.S.W.	Stephanie Smith, M.S.
Amy A. Jarzebowicz, M.S.	

Todays date: _____

COVER PAGE: Medical-Genetic Family History Questionnaire

You are being asked to provide family history information at a time that we know is difficult for you; however, this information may be important at some point in providing medical care for your child. There are many medical conditions that can run in families. We are trying to obtain a complete medical history because your child may need this information in the future. Please answer the questions as best as you can. If you have any questions about how to answer anything, please ask your adoption worker for help. Each birth parent should complete a Medical-Genetic Family History Form.

This page contains information that is needed for the child's records. It will be shared with the child or the adoptive parents *only* if you sign a special sheet giving your permission to release this information for their use.

Child's Name: _____
                    Last   First   Middle

Date of Birth: _____

Birthplace: Please Circle: Hospital   Home   Other _____

Provide name and address of birth location as well as the name of the doctor or health worker who delivered the baby:

_____
_____

Birth Mother's Name: _____
                           Last   First   Middle

Date of Birth: _____

Current Permanent Mailing Address:

_____

Birth Father's Name: _____
                          Last   First   Middle

Date of Birth: _____

Current Permanent Mailing Address:

_____

Case Identification Number: _____

Name and Address of Agency involved in the Adoption: _____

_____

PREGNANCY CARE WITH THIS CHILD   Agency #_____   Today's date _____   p. 1 of 1

In what month of your pregnancy did you first see a health care worker? ___ 1 mo ___ 2 mos
___ 3 mos ___ 4 mos ___ 5 mos ___6 mos ___ 7 mos ___ 8 mos ___ 9 mos ___ no prenatal care

Did you have, or were you exposed to, any of the following in pregnancy?

	Yes	No	Don't Know	What Months In Pregnancy?	If Yes, Please Explain
Fever (101 degrees or over)	__	__	__	_____	_____
Rashes	__	__	__	_____	_____
Infection	__	__	__	_____	_____
X-rays/radiation	__	__	__	_____	_____
Chemicals	__	__	__	_____	_____
Toxic/hazardous wastes	__	__	__	_____	_____
Sexually transmitted diseases	__	__	__	_____	_____
HIV/AIDS	__	__	__	_____	_____
Diabetes	__	__	__	_____	_____
Measles (or rubella)	__	__	__	_____	_____
Mumps or chicken pox	__	__	__	_____	_____
High blood pressure	__	__	__	_____	_____
Toxemia	__	__	__	_____	_____

Did you take any of the following? If yes, when in pregnancy, and how much per week did you take?

	Yes	No	Don't Know	What Months In Pregnancy?	How Much Per Week?
Alcohol (include beer and wine)	__	__	__	_____	_____
Cigarettes	__	__	__	_____	_____
Cocaine/crack (circle)	__	__	__	_____	_____
Heroin/Methadone (circle)	__	__	__	_____	_____
LSD/acid	__	__	__	_____	_____
Marijuana/pot	__	__	__	_____	_____
Amphetamines (uppers)	__	__	__	_____	_____
Barbiturates (downers)	__	__	__	_____	_____
Others (specify)___	__	__	__	_____	_____

Did you take any of the following medications? If yes, name the medication, and explain when and how much was taken during the pregnancy.

	Yes	No	Don't Know	What Months In Pregnancy?	Name of Medication/ How Much Per Week?
Prescription medicines	__	__	__	_____	_____
	__	__	__	_____	_____
	__	__	__	_____	_____
Over the counter medications	__	__	__	_____	_____
	__	__	__	_____	_____
	__	__	__	_____	_____
Seizure medications	__	__	__	_____	_____
	__	__	__	_____	_____
	__	__	__	_____	_____
Other _____	__	__	__	_____	_____

Did you have any genetic tests in pregnancy? ___ Yes ___ No ___ Don't Know If Yes, please explain_____

DELIVERY AND BIRTH INFORMATION OF THE CHILD Agency #____ Date _____ p. 1 of 2

How many hours were you in labor? _____ *The delivery was:* _____ Vaginal _____ Cesarean

If cesarean, why? _____

Were there any problems during this delivery? ____ Yes ____ No ____ Don't Know
If Yes, please explain _____

The baby was born ____ Breech ____ Head first ____ Don't Know

Was there a heart murmur at birth? ____Yes ____ No ____ Don't Know
If Yes, specify the cardiac diagnosis_____

Were any other problems noted AT birth? ____ Yes ____ No ____ Don't Know
If Yes, please explain _____
_____

Were any other problems noted AFTER birth? ___ Yes ___ No ____ Don't Know
If Yes, please explain, and indicate the age of the child when the problem was noted _____
_____

A child whose parents are related by blood may have a higher chance of having health problems. For this reason, we need to know if there is any blood relationship between the birth parents. *If this child's parents are related by blood* please check off the relationship in the list below:

____ Father/daughter ____ Mother/son ____ Brother/sister ____ Half brother/sister
____ Uncle/niece ____ Aunt/nephew ____ Cousin ____ Other (please explain)

BIRTH AND MEDICAL INFORMATION FOR THIS CHILD

Sex of child: ____ Male ____ Female *Date of Birth:* _____ *Time of Birth:* _____

Hospital of birth: _____ *City:* _____ *State:* _____ *County:*_____

The baby was born: ____ At Term Premature at ____ weeks Postmature at ____weeks

Birth weight: _____ lbs. _____ oz. *Birth length:* _____ inches

APGAR score: _____ At one minute _____ At five minutes _____ Don't Know

Baby's blood type: __ A __ B __ AB __ O *Rh factor:* __ Positive __ Negative __ Don't Know

Were any of the following newborn screening tests positive?

	Yes	No	Don't Know
Cystic fibrosis			
Galactosemia			
Hypothyroidism			
PKU (phenylketonuria)			
Sickle cell disease			
Maple syrup urine disease			
Other (specify) _____			

Has the child had any genetic testing? ____ Yes ____ No ____Don't Know If Yes, please explain_____

Date: _____ Medical-Genetic Family Hx (circle): Birth Mother Birth Father Agency# _____ p. 1 of 8

Medical-Genetic Family History Questionnaire

Please supply the following information about yourself:

Your year of birth: _____ *Are you adopted?* ___Yes ___No ___Don't Know

Ethnic Background (circle all that apply): White   Jewish   African American
Hispanic Origin Native American   Asian   Pacific Islander   Other (Please list):
_____

Highest grade completed (circle): 1 2 3 4 5 6 7 8 9 10 11 12 13 14 15 16 17+

Were you ever in special classes to provide extra help in learning? ___ Yes   ___No

Have you had any major illnesses? ___Yes ___No

If yes, please explain: _____

Do you have, or have you had, any mental illness? ___ Yes ____ No

If yes, please explain:_____

Have you ever been told that you have a genetic/inherited disease? ____ Yes
____No

If yes, please explain:_____

Have you ever been told that you are a carrier of a genetic/inherited disease?
___ Yes ___No

If yes, what disease? _____

*Print the first names and descriptions of all of your children (i.e., the child's broth-
ers and sisters). List in order of birth, including children who have died. If a child
died, please indicate age at death and the cause of death.*

First Name	Relationship to the present child (full, half, or step)	Date of Birth	Health Problems
1. _____	_____	_____	_____
2. _____	_____	_____	_____
3. _____	_____	_____	_____
4. _____	_____	_____	_____
5. _____	_____	_____	_____
6. _____	_____	_____	_____

Have you (or your partner) had any miscarriages? ____ Yes (How many?) _____
No_____

Date: _____ Medical-Genetic Family Hx (circle): Birth Mother Birth Father Agency# ___ p. 2 of 8

YOUR BROTHERS AND SISTERS

How many living brothers do you have? _____

Do you have any brothers who died? ___ Yes (list each below)   ___ No

Age at Death	Cause of Death	Medical Problem involved in the cause of death, if known
_____	_____	_____
_____	_____	_____
_____	_____	_____

Have any of your brothers had any serious health, physical, mental or learning problems?

_____ Yes   _____ No   _____ Don't Know

If yes, please explain:_____

How many living sisters do you have? _____

Do you have any sisters who died? ___ Yes (list each below)   ___ No

Age at Death	Cause of Death	Medical Problem involved in the cause of death, if known
_____	_____	_____
_____	_____	_____
_____	_____	_____

Have any of your sisters had any serious health, physical, mental or learning problems?

_____ Yes   _____ No   _____ Don't Know

If yes, please explain:_____

Do any of your brothers or sisters have a different father or mother? If yes, please indicate which brother or sister, and which parent was different from yours:

_____

YOUR PARENTS

In what year was your mother born? _____

Has she had any serious health, physical, mental or learning problems?

___Yes ___No ___Don't Know

If yes, please explain: _____

_____

*If she has died, cause of death and age:*_____

Highest grade she completed in school (circle): 1 2 3 4 5 6 7 8 9 10 11 12 13 14 15 16 17+

Did she receive special education? ___ Yes ___ No ___Don't Know

Date: _____   Medical-Genetic Family Hx (circle): Birth Mother Birth Father Agency# ____ p. 3 of 8

*In what year was your father born?*_____

Has he had any serious health, physical, mental or learning problems? ___Yes ___No ___Don't Know

If yes, please explain: _____

If he has died, cause of death and age: _____

Highest grade he completed in school (circle): 1 2 3 4 5 6 7 8 9 10 11 12 13 14 15 16 17+

Was he ever in special classes to provide extra help in learning? ___Yes ___ No ___Don't Know

YOUR GRANDPARENTS

Your Mother's Mother:

Has she had any serious health, physical, mental or learning problems? ___Yes ___No ___Don't Know

If yes, please explain:_____

If she has died, cause of death and age: _____

Country of origin of her ancestors (for example, Italy, Scotland, etc.): _____

Ethnic Background (circle all that apply): White, Jewish, African American, Hispanic Origin, Native American, Asian, Pacific Islander, Other (Please list): _____

Your Mother's Father:

Has he had any serious health, physical, mental or learning problems? ___Yes ___ No ___Don't Know

If yes, please explain: _____

If he has died, cause of death and age: _____

Country of origin of his ancestors (for example, Italy, Scotland, etc.): _____

Ethnic Background (circle all that apply): White, Jewish, African American, Hispanic Origin, Native American, Asian, Pacific Islander, Other (Please list): _____

Your Father's Mother:

Has she had any serious health, physical, mental or learning problems? ___Yes ___No ___Don't Know

If yes, please explain: _____

If she has died, cause of death and age: _____

Country of origin of her ancestors (for example, Italy, Scotland, etc.): _____

Ethnic Background (circle all that apply): White, Jewish, African American, Hispanic Origin, Native American, Asian, Pacific Islander, Other (Please list): _____

Your Father's Father:

Has he had any serious health, physical, mental, or learning problems? ___Yes ___No ___Don't Know

If yes, please explain: _____

If he has died, cause of death and age: _____

Country of origin of his ancestors (for example, Italy, Scotland, etc.): _____

Ethnic Background (circle all that apply): White, Jewish, African American, Hispanic Origin, Native American, Asian, Pacific Islander, Other (Please list):

Date: _____   Medical-Genetic Family Hx (circle): Birth Mother Birth Father Agency# ___ p. 4 of 8

Genetic-Medical History

Check "Yes" or "No" if you or any of your blood relatives (i.e., your parents, grand-parents, aunts, uncles, brothers, sisters, cousins, nieces and nephews) ever had, or now have, any of the medical conditions listed. Include only relatives who are your blood relatives (omit relatives related by marriage or adoption, but include half brothers and half sisters).

	Yourself		*Blood relative*		*How related*
Specific Medical Conditions	*Yes*	*No*	*Yes*	*No*	*to you?*
1. *Blindness or other visual problems (note age affected)*					
2. *Cataracts (note age affected)*					
3. *Glaucoma (note age affected)*					
4. *Deafness, hearing difficulties (note age affected)*					
5. *Unusual shape or missing ear*					
6. *Speech problems*					
8. *Dental problems Example - extra or missing teeth*					
9. *Cleft lip (harelip)*					
10. *Cleft palate*					
11. *Learning disability (slow learner)*					
12. *Mental retardation (estimate severity)*					
13. *Attention deficit disorder and/or hyperactivity*					
14. *Down syndrome*					
15. *Other chromosome abnormality (please specify)*					
16. *Schizophrenia (note age affected)*					
17. *Bipolar depression (note age affected)*					

If you answered yes to any of the above, please complete the following:

Number (from above)	Age when first affected	Relationship to the child	Comments (name of disorder if known)

Date: _____   Medical-Genetic Family Hx (circle): Birth Mother Birth Father Agency# ___ p. 5 of 8

Specific Medical Conditions	Yourself Yes	Yourself No	Blood relative Yes	Blood relative No	How related to you?
18. *Other mental illness (please specify)*					
19. *Hydrocephalus (water on the brain)*					
20. *Microcephaly (small head)*					
21. *Birthmarks (please describe)* *Example - unusual shape, size, or number*					
22. *Patches of hair of different color*					
23. *Patches of skin of different color* *Example - white or brown spots*					
24. *Skin problems* *Severe eczema, acne, or other*					
25. *Bleeding problems or hemophilia*					
26. *Sickle cell disease*					
27. *Thalassemia*					
28. *High blood pressure (hyypertension) (specify age)*					
29. *Kidney problems (specify age)*					
30. *Stroke (specify age)*					
31. *Heart attack (specify age)*					
32. *Born with heart defect* *Example - hole in heart*					
33. *Born with open spine (spina bifida)*					
34. *Born with missing brain (anencephaly)*					
35. *Born with hip problems (dislocated hips)*					

If you answered yes to any of the above, please complete the following:

Number (from above)	Age when first affected	Relationship to the child	Comments (name of disorder if known)

Date: _____ Medical-Genetic Family Hx (circle): Birth Mother Birth Father Agency# ___ p. 6 of 8

Specific Medical Conditions	Yourself Yes	No	Blood relative Yes	No	How related to you?
36. *Dwarfism or short stature*					
37. *Spinal curvature (scoliosis)*					
38. *Unusually formed bones or many broken bones*					
39. *Unusually formed hands (please describe)* Example - extra/missing/webbed fingers					
40. *Unusually formed feet (please describe)* Example - extra/missing/webbed toes					
41. *Club foot*					
42. *Other birth defects (please specify)* (not listed above)					
43. *Arthritis, joint problems (specify age)*					
44. *Muscular dystrophy (age affected and type if known)*					
45. *Muscle weakness (note age affected)*					
46. *Loss of muscle control (note age affected)*					
47. *Pyloric stenosis (projectile vomiting)*					
48. *Breast cancer (age diagnosed)*					
49. *Colon cancer (age diagnosed)*					
50. *Ovarian cancer (age diagnosed)*					
51. *Other cancers (please specify type and age diagnosed) (include childhood cancers)*					
52. *Cystic fibrosis*					
53. *Alzheimer disease (note age affected)*					
54. *Dementia (note age affected) (mental deterioration)*					

If you answered yes to any of the above, please complete the following:

Number (from above)	Age when first affected	Relationship to the child	Comments (name of disorder if known)

Specific Medical Conditions	Yourself Yes	Yourself No	Blood relative Yes	Blood relative No	How related to you?
55. Huntington disease (chorea) (note age affected)					
56. Neurofibromatosis					
57. Multiple sclerosis (note age affected)					
58. Tay sachs disease					
59. Cerebral palsy					
60. Seizures, convulsions, epilepsy (note age affected and type if known)					
61. Adult diabetes (specify age) (insulin or non-insulin dependent)					
62. Childhood diabetes (specify age)					
63. Thyroid disorder (specify if under-active or over-active)					
64. Kidney problems (note age affected)					
65. Respiratory or breathing problems (specify age) Example - emphysema					
66. Asthma					
67. Allergies - hay fever (pollen)					
68. Allergies - food (please specify)					
69. Allergies - medicine (please specify)					
70. Chemical dependency (alcohol)					
71. Chemical dependency -other drugs (please specify)					
72. Weight problems (obesity or anorexia)					

If you answered yes to any of the above, please complete the following:

Number (from above)	Age when first affected	Relationship to the child	Comments (name of disorder if known)

Date: _____ Medical-Genetic Family Hx (circle): Birth Mother Birth Father Agency# ___ p. 8 of 8

Specific Medical Conditions	*Yourself*		*Blood relative*		*How related to you?*
	Yes	*No*	*Yes*	*No*	
73. *Infertility*					
74. *Miscarriages* If yes, how many?					
75. *Stillbirths* If yes, how many?					
76. *Neonatal deaths* (died before one month old)					
77. *Infant deaths* (died before one year of age)					
78. *Childhood deaths (specify age and cause)*					
79. *HIV (Human Immunodeficiency Virus)*					
80. *AIDS (Acquired Immunodeficiency Syndrome)*					
81. *Frequent Infections (Immune deficiency)*					

If you answered yes to any of the above, please complete the following:

Number (from above)	Age when first affected	Relationship to the child	Comments (name of disorder if known)

Has anyone in the family had any genetic testing? Please explain:

_____

_____

_____

_____

Is there anything else you think we should know about you or your family?

_____

_____

_____

_____

APPENDIX *A.5*

The Genetics Library

The following is an annotated list of my recommendations for medical genetics books, pedigree drawing programs, and Internet resources for the clinician seeking to supplement his or her personal or medical center library. I provide the size of the books and their approximate costs to give an idea of the scope and affordability of the reference.

PEDIGREE SOFTWARE DRAWING PROGRAMS

To date, the available programs are most useful for preparing pedigrees for publication, keeping track of evaluations on large families, or collecting pedigrees for research. Both *Cyrillic* and *Progeny* are excellent for storing clinical and molecular data in relation to pedigree information. They are somewhat cumbersome for everyday clinical practice. Both programs use standardized pedigree nomenclature. *Cyrillic* includes a program for calculating breast cancer risks from the Claus model.

Cyrillic (Version 2.0), cost ~$500–$600
Contact information: Cherwell Scientific Publishing, 744 Antonio Road, Suite 27 A, Palo Alto, CA 94303, Phone (415) 852-0720, E-mail csp.usa@cherwell.com, URL: http://www.cherwell.com
System Requirements: IBM PC or Compatible running Windows 3.1, Windows 95, or Windows NT with 4 MB RAM.
Comments: A free on-line discussion group is helpful for the snafus one is bound to encounter with any software program!

Progeny (Windows or Mac version), cost ~$900 (Recommended for use with a 486 DX 66 MHZ processor with 12 MB of RAM, or Pentium processor with 16 MB, and 15" SVGA monitor)
Contact Information: Progeny Software, LLC, 1025 Widener Lane, South Bend, IN

46614. Telephone (219) 299-4900, FAX (219) 299-1601, E-mail @proge-ny2000.com, URL: http://www.progeny2000.com

GenoSketch This is a shareware program developed by Alan Farmer (E-mail farmer@netaxs.com) that is still in process, but looks promising! It is intended for clinical use in drawing pedigrees. Additional program features can be added for a small fee. URL: http://www.netaxs.com/~farmer/gsketch/

INTERNET RESOURCES

OMIM (On-line Mendelian Inheritance in Man)

> http://www3.ncbi.nlm.nih.gov/omim/searchomim.html

This site is a unique Web resource and often is the first place to turn for information about a particular genetic issue. It is an extensive database of inherited disorders, maintained by the Johns Hopkins University School of Medicine providing information on genetic syndromes, clinical presentation, cytogenetics, genetic mapping, pathogenesis, and population genetics. There are hypertext links to the National Library of Medicine's MEDLINE database.

European Directory of DNA Laboratories (EDDNAL)

> http://www.eddnal.com/

An extensive directory of the DNA laboratories in Europe.

Helix

> http://www.genetests.org

Helix is an international directory of diagnostic and research laboratories providing molecular genetic testing for a variety of genetic diseases. The site is funded by the National Library of Medicine and Maternal and Child Health Bureau, and maintained by the University of Washington. The database is accessible by obtaining a password (application available on-line). The laboratories are self-listed. There are useful hypertext links to International listings of clinical genetics service providers.

GeneClinics

> http://www.geneclinics.org

This electronic textbook contains expert-authored clinical information relating genetic testing to the diagnosis, management, and counseling of individuals and families with inherited disorders. It is funded by the National Library of Medicine and the National Human Genome Research Institute of the National Institute of Health and maintained by the University of Washington in Seattle. Links to information about genetic counseling service providers are given.

Information For Genetics Professionals

http://www.kumc.edu/gec/geneinfo.html

If you only "bookmark" one genetic Web site, this is the one! This Web site is up-dated on a regular basis by genetic counselor, Debra Collins, MS, at University of Kansas Medical Center. Collins maintains an extremely comprehensive listing of clinical genetic resources, pedigree drawing programs, family support information, and on-line databases. The site has many useful hyperlinks.

Online Resource Center (Genetics Education and Counseling Program, University of Pittsburgh, Dept. Human Genetics)

http://www.pitt.edu/~edugene/resource/

Intended as an on-line resource for genetic counselors, this Web site has links to a wealth of information on a variety of practical topics related to genetic services (e.g., education and teaching resources, books and journals, ethics, news topics, lab information, support groups).

CDC Office of Genetics & Disease Prevention Home Page

http://www.cdc.gov/genetics/

This regularly updated Web site provides access to current information on the im-pact of human genetic research and the Human Genome Project on public health and disease prevention. You can register for their on-line newsletter that includes headlines from the past week's news and highlights scientific publications, upcom-ing events, and Web sites that are relevant to genetics and public heatlh.

National Genome Research Institute

http://www.nhgri.nigh.gov/

This is the Web site for the Human Genome Project. It includes information about the Center for Inherited Disease Research, ELSI (Ethical, Legal and Social Implica-tions), a schedule of workshops and conferences, and timely topics in the news. My favorite section is a glossary of genetic terms that allows the user to download audio and video files.

Gene Letter

http://www.geneletter.org

An on-line newsletter about new and controversial issues in genetics

NORD (National Organization for Rare Disorders)

http://www.rarediseases.org

A network of organizations representing individuals with rare disorders. Includes a networking program for individuals and families.

March of Dimes Homepage

http://modimes.org

General information about birth defects and their prevention, and a resource list of fact sheets on genetic disorders in English and Spanish.

Alliance of Genetic Support Groups

http://www.geneticalliance.org

This is an outstanding resource for finding support groups and lay literature for individuals with genetic disorders. The toll-free helpline is 1-800-336-GENE.

Family Village—A Global Community of Disability-Related Resources

http://www.familyvillage.wisc.edu/

An easy to navigate site, for parents of children with mental retardation and other disabilities, providing medical information and resources for a variety of inherited disorders.

National Institute of Neurological Disorders and Stroke (NINDS)

http://www.ninds.nih.gov/

Grouped by neurological conditions, this database provides a brief general description of the disease, its treatment, prognosis, research, and available support groups. In depth references for health professionals are included.

Genetics Information-National Cancer Institute

http://cancernet.nci.nih.gov/p_genetics.html

This site is part of the National Cancer Institute's main on-line information center for patients and physicians. It has several basic monographs on genetic testing as well as position statements about testing by groups such as the American College of Medical Genetics, the American Society of Human Genetics, and the American Society of Clinical Oncologists. A wonderful resource is the ability to query the database to locate a board-certified or eligible genetic counselor.

Lahey Hitchcock Cancer Risk Assessment Clinic

http://www.lahey.org

This URL connects you to the general web page for the Lahey Hitchcock Clinic in Massachusetts. You can then search under genetics to find a clear and comprehensive discussion about genetic testing and counseling for breast cancer. A listing of centers around the country that offer genetic counseling for cancer risk assessment is a valuable resource.

The Genetics of Cancer

http://www.cancergenetics.org/

This site, developed by the Robert H. Lurie Cancer Center at Northwestern University Medical School, provides basic and clinical information on new advances in cancer genetics, case studies, and specific information for primary care physicians and nurse practitioners.

Wisconsin Stillbirth Service Program (WiSSP)

http://www.wisc.edu/wissp

A Web site containing the standard of care for the genetic evaluation of a stillbirth (clinical evaluation, photographs, autopsy, chromosomes, radiographs, pre/perinatal history, and Kleihuaer-Betke testing)

Kathryn and Alan C. Greenberg Center for Skeletal Dysplasias

http://www.med.jhu.edu/Greenberg.Center/Greenbrg.htm

An informative Web site with clinical summaries of multiple skeletal dysplasias as well as an on-line opportunity to "ask the experts" questions about the diagnosis and management of skeletal dysplasias.

CD-ROM

POSSUM 5.0, New subscribers cost ~$2000

Contact information: Developed by Professor David Danks and Dr. Agnes Bankier at the Murdoch Institute and the Victorian Clinical Genetics Services at the Royal Children's Hospital Melbourne.

For more information contact The Murdoch Institute, Royal Children's Hospital, Flemington Road, Parkville, Victoria 3052, Australia. Phone: +61 3 9345 5045; FAX: + 61 3 9348 1391. URL: http://murdoch.rch.unimelb.edu.au/possum.htm

Comments: Possum is a software tool, using a multimedia format including pictures, X-rays, diagrams, histopathology and video clips, to assist clinicians in syndrome diagnosis in their patients. More than 2500 syndromes are included.

The following are available from Electronic Publishing, Oxford University Press, 200 Madison Avenue, New York, NY 10016. Phone (212) 726-6000, FAX (212) 725-2972.

- *London Dysmorphology Database,* cost ~$850. DOS-based database and CD-ROM for Win95 (1996 version 2.0) A database by Robin Winter and Michael Baraitser with close to 3000 syndromes. Note the CD-ROM with clinical photographs is purchased separately.

- *London Neurogenetics Database,* cost ~$850. More than 2600 syndromes involving the central and peripheral nervous system with a review of the neurological features, neuroradiology, neurophysiology, neuropathology, and nerve and muscle biopsy findings. Note the CD-ROM with clinical photographs is purchased separately.

- *Human Cytogenetics Database,* cost ~$700. Clinical and cytogenetic data on more than 1200 chromosomal aneuploidies, developed by Albert Schinzel. Note the CD-ROM with clinical photographs is purchased separately.
- *Dysmorphology Photo Library,* cost $695. This is a library of more than 10,000 clinical photographs to illustrate syndromes in the London Dysmorphology Database or the London Neurogenetics Database.

BOOKS (for those of us who prefer the old-fashioned library)

General Inherited Disease References

Clarke JTR (1996). *A Clinical Guide To Inherited Metabolic Diseases.* Cambridge: Cambridge University Press, 280 pp., cost ~$50 cloth, $18 paperback
   Although this book can hardly replace Scriver and colleagues' *Metabolic and Molecular Bases of Inherited Disease* (see below), it is a concise and practical clinical approach to inherited metabolic disorders (and a heck of a lot easier to cart to clinic). I find the approach by symptomatology (such as how to evaluate acute metabolic illness in a newborn) and laboratory investigation particularly useful.

Gardner RJM, Sutherland GR (1996). *Chromosome Abnormalities and Genetic Counseling,* 2nd ed. New York, Oxford: Oxford University Press, 478 pp., cost ~$60
   An indispensable book for obstetricians and pediatricians who are involved in the diagnosis of fetuses and newborns with chromosome abnormalities. The sections on prenatal diagnosis are particularly useful.

Hall JG, Froster-Iskenius UG, Allanson JE (1989). *Handbook of Normal Physical Measurements.* Oxford: Oxford University Press, 504 pp., cost ~$54
   To appreciate the unusual, one must first appreciate the usual. This is a useful reference on how to take measurements to evaluate children and adults with dysmorphic features and/or structural anomalies. Normal measurements are not adjusted for ethnic variables. It includes the "hows" and "whats" of measuring humans. Included are normal growth charts for several common syndromes such as Down syndrome, William syndrome, Marfan syndrome, and Turner syndrome.

King RA, Rotter JI, Motulsky AG (eds) (1992). *The Genetic Basis of Common Diseases.* New York: Oxford University Press, 978 pp., cost ~$150
   I am eager to see the new edition of this book, which is due in 1999. A whirlwind of advances has occurred in this field since the original publication. I am confidant that the new edition will be even more informative than the first.

Rimoin DL, Connor JM, Pyeritz RE (eds) (1996). *Emery and Rimoin's Principles and Practice of Medical Genetics,* 3rd ed. New York: Churchill Livingstone, 2937 pp. (2 volumes), cost ~$310
   Another classic volume for the genetics library. A nice resource for overviews of broad topics in medical genetics such as mental retardation, deafness, an approach

to the dysmorphic child, carrier screening, etc. A new edition should be in print in 2000.

Scriver CR, Beaudet AL, Sly WS, Valle D (eds) (1995). *The Metabolic and Molecular Bases of Inherited Disease,* New York: McGraw-Hill, Inc, 4605 pp. (3 volumes), cost ~$325, available in CD-ROM ~$345.

Although you must be a weight lifter to carry these three hefty volumes to clinic, this tome is in every genetics professional's collection. Individuals without a firm foundation in genetics may have difficulty wading through some of the chapters. The volumes cover many disorders that are not traditionally considered metabolic diseases (such as fragile X syndrome). A new edition is pending.

Vogel F, Motulsky AG (1996). *Human Genetics,* 3rd ed. Berlin, Heidelberg, New York: Springer-Verlag, 851 pp., cost ~$99

This is a classic text in the theories and practices of human genetics. Although it draws on clinical examples, this is not light reading for the average clinician; yet it is required reading for anyone wanting a good foundation for critical review of research in human genetics.

Brief (and Reasonably Priced) Overviews of Medical Genetics

Connor M, Ferguson-Smith M (1997). *Essential Medical Genetics,* 5th ed. Oxford: Blackwell Scientific, 236 pp., cost ~$40

The title is a good description for the book's contents; here's what you need to know for a practical, clinical approach to human genetics. A helpful synthesis of overall principles with specific syndromes.

Robinson A, Linden MG (1993). *Clinical Genetics Handbook,* 2nd ed. Boston: Blackwell Scientific Publications, 614 pp., cost ~$45

Although this book is another that is in dire need of a new edition, it is still a useful clinical handbook for a general overview of common genetic disorders by system. Each chapter includes a general overview of the disease or problem, clinical notes, procedures for diagnostic confirmation, considerations in management, psychosocial and educational components, and disease specific resources. I still use it for looking up empirical risks for general conditions, psychiatric disorders, mental retardation, and hearing loss.

James JL (ed) (1998). *Principles of Molecular Medicine.* New Jersey: Humana Press, 1056 pp., cost ~$175

One of the first books to link the emerging principles of molecular medicine to the major clinical aspects of medicine, including diagnostics, pathophysiology and new therapeutic avenues.

Lashley FRC (1998). *Clinical Genetics in Nursing Practice,* 2nd ed. New York: Springer Publishing Company, 543 pp., cost ~$80

A comprehensive overview of the nursing issues related to the counseling and management of individuals with genetic disorders. Unfortunately this book does not use standardized pedigree symbols.

Lea DH, Jenkins JF, Francomano CA (1998). *Genetics in Clinical Practice: New Direction for Nursing and Health Care.* Boston: Jones and Bartlett Publishers, Inc., 300 pp., cost ~$42
   A good investment for nurses interested in summary of clinical genetics that is relevant to their practice. The authors use case studies to illustrate points.

Seashore MR, Wappner RS (1996). *Genetics in Primary Care and Clinical Medicine.* Stamford: Appelton & Lange, 334 pp., cost ~$35
   The organization of this overview of medical genetics by disease system is a practical approach. There are useful summary tables providing practical information and good clinical illustrations.

Thompson MW, McInnes RR, Willard HF (1991). *Thompson & Thompson Genetics in Medicine,* 5th ed. Philadelphia: W. B. Saunders, 500 pp., cost ~$46
   I hesitate to include this because it is sorely in need of a new edition. It is still one the best reviews of clinical genetics, but information about testing and classifications for many diseases needs updating.

Genetic Counseling

Baker DL, Schuette JL, Uhlmann WR (ed) (1998). *A Guide To Genetic Counseling.* New York: Wiley-Liss, 416 pp., cost ~$75 cloth, $43 paper
   Intended to be used as a textbook for training genetic counseling students, this book provides everything you ever wanted to know about genetic counseling and *needed* to ask. Case examples are provided to illustrate the skills, techniques, and principles presented throughout the book.

Fisher NL (ed) (1996). *Cultural and Ethnic Diversity. A Guide for Genetics Professionals.* Baltimore and London: Johns Hopkins University Press, 246 pp., cost ~$45
   This is a comprehensive and unique summary of the many aspects to consider when providing genetic assessment to individuals from varying cultural backgrounds living in the United States. Knowing this information is helpful when trying to obtain family and medical history information from clients of diverse backgrounds, although it is important not to stereotype any individual based on his or her cultural/ethnic background. Cultural groups that are covered include Amish, Deaf, Anglo-Saxon, Christian, Latino, African American, Southwest Native Americans, Chinese, Japanese, Southeast Asian, Korean, and Asian Indian.

Greenwood Genetic Center *(1995). Counseling Aids for Geneticists,* 3rd ed. Available from Greenwood Genetic Center, 1-(800) 473-9411, cost ~$35
   This spiral-bound book contains 73 simple illustrations of basic patterns of in-

heritance, karyotypes of common chromosome anomalies, and examples of prenatal diagnostic techniques to be used as a visual aid for providing genetic counseling.

Harper PS (1998). *Practical Genetic Counseling,* 4th ed. Oxford: Butterworth Heinemann Limited, 364 pp., cost ~$67

This is a handy reference of general recurrence risks and genetic counseling issues for a variety of common disorders.

Dysmorphology and Anomalies of the Head, Face, and Neck

Buyse ML (1990). *Birth Defects Encyclopedia: The Comprehensive, Systematic, Illustrated Reference Source for the Diagnosis, Delineation, Etiology, Biodynamics, Occurrence, Prevention, and Treatment of Human Anomalies of Clinical Relevance.* Dover: Blackwell Scientific Publications, Inc., 1892 pp., cost ~$275.

The title summarizes the contents. Like any encyclopedia, this book provides limited facts on many conditions. The book was printed when molecular testing was available for only a few conditions so the information is out-of-date for many diseases.

Cohen MM (1997). *The Child with Multiple Birth Defects.* Oxford University Press: Oxford. 267 pp., cost ~$82

Cohen provides an easy to follow approach to "syndromology" and teratology for evaluation of the fetus or child with multiple congenital anomalies.

Gorlin RJ, Cohen MM, Levin LS (1990). *Syndromes of the Head and Neck,* 3rd ed. New York: Oxford University Press, 977 pp., cost ~$263

Despite its age, this book is still a classic tool in syndromic diagnosis of individuals with unusual facial features. The combination of system oriented clinical descriptions with black-and-white photographs plus an excellent index make this book indispensable for a genetics clinic.

Jones KL (1997). *Smith's Recognizable Patterns of Human Malformation,* 5th ed. Philadelphia: W. B. Saunders, 857 pp., cost ~$65

This is the bible of genetic dysmorphologists. A short disease synopsis is combined with a picture for each condition. The appendix is a guide for differential diagnosis by pattern of anomaly (for example, disorders with enamel hypoplasia, or conditions with colobomata of iris).

Tewfik TL, Der Kaloustian VM (eds) (1997). *Congenital Anomalies of the Ear, Nose and Throat.* New York: Oxford University Press, 579 pp., cost ~$197

With an orientation toward surgical management of these conditions, the editors provide extensive tables of the hundreds of hereditary ENT syndromes. This approach is useful for determining a differential diagnosis but I found myself turning to other sources to get a better "feel" for the syndromes.

Wiedemann H-R, Kunze J (1997). *Clinical Syndromes,* 3rd ed. Italy: Times Mirror International Publishers Limited, 684 pp., cost ~$150

This authorized translation of the fourth German language edition, "Atlas der Klinischen Syndrome," provides short summaries of many inherited disorders with multiple pictures (including radiographic findings) of the syndromes on the facing page. The organization of the contents by the presenting sign or symptoms (e.g., syndromes with prominent anomalies of the cranium, face, or both; syndromes with tall stature as a prominent feature) is extremely valuable.

Detection of Fetal Anomalies by Ultrasound

Sanders RC (ed), Blackmon LR, Hogge WA, Wulfsberg EA (assistant eds) (1996). *Structural Fetal Abnormalties: The Total Picture.* St. Louis: Mosby, 284 pp., cost ~$63

This book is to obstetricians, geneticists, genetic counselors, sonographers, obstetrical nurses, and nurse-midwives what "Smith's Recognizable Malformation" is to dysmorphologists. Sanders et al. provide an integrated approach for diagnosing and managing fetal problems identified by ultrasound. Each condition (e.g. pleural effusion, polyhydramnios, intracranial teratoma) is divided into discussions of epidemiology/genetics, sonography findings and differential diagnosis, pregnancy management, neonatology, and surgery (if appropriate). Appendices of differential diagnoses of abnormal in utero sonographic findings and of the sonographic features of unusual congenital syndromes are extremely useful.

Snijders RJM, Nicholaides KH (1996). *Ultrasound Markers for Fetal Chromosomal Defects.* New York: Parthenon Publishing Group, 200 pp., cost ~$65

Another important book for health professionals involved in the diagnosis and management of fetal anomalies.

Taybi Hooshang, Lachman RS (1996). *Radiology of Syndromes, Metabolic Disorders, and Skeletal Dysplasias,* 4th ed. St Louis: Mosby, 1135 pp., cost ~$225

Brief summaries of the pathology, clinical and radiological manifestations, and differential diagnosis of close to 1000 conditions. The disorders are reviewed in alphabetical order under the broad categories of syndromes, metabolic disorders, and skeletal dysplasias.

Deafness

Gorlin RJ, Toriello HV, MM Cohen (1995). *Hereditary Hearing Loss and Its Syndromes.* New York and Oxford: Oxford University Press, 457 pp., cost ~$262

A classic reference for genetic diagnosis of individuals with hearing loss. The text is nicely complemented with photographs and a comprehensive reference list for further reading. The index is a great resource for compiling a differential diagnosis. Major molecular advances in hearing loss have been made since publication but this still does not detract from the usefulness of the text.

Also see Tewfik and Der Kaloustian (under) Dysmorphology above.

Eye Disorders

Traboulsi EI (1998). *Genetic Diseases of the Eye.* Oxford: Oxford University Press, 512 pp., cost ~$215

A comprehensive sourcebook on genetic eye diseases reviewing the history, pathogenesis, etiology, epidemiology, classification, clinical manifestations, diagnosis, treatment, and molecular advances for many conditions.

Immune Disorders

Ochs HD, Smith E, Puck J (eds) (1998). *Genetics of Primary Immunodeficiency Diseases.* Oxford: Oxford University Press, 624 pp., cost ~$140

A groundbreaking book bridging the gap between the basic and clinical sciences of immunologic genetics. A particularly useful book for allergists, infectious disease specialists, hematologists, and oncologists.

Neurological

Baraitser M (1997). *The Genetics of Neurological Disorders,* 3rd ed. Oxford: Oxford University Press, 443 pp., cost ~$90

Baraitser provides brief overviews of the hereditary basis for neurological disorders. It is most useful for clinicians who already have a familiarity with most of the features of these disorders; others might find they need to turn to other references for more detailed descriptions of the conditions.

Emery AEH (1998). *Neuromuscular Disorders: Clinical and Medical Genetics.* New York: Wiley-Liss, 450 pp., cost ~$120.

Emery, an authority on this rapidly changing topic, provides a comprehensive overview of neuromuscular disorders. Disorders are discussed by clinical features, pathology, inheritance, molecular genetics, screening, prenatal diagnosis, prevention and counseling, and possible treatments by drug and gene therapy.

Renal Disorders

Morgan S, Grunfeld J-P (eds) (1998). *Inherited Disorders of the Kidney.* Oxford: Oxford University Press. 648 pp., cost ~$199

A practical approach to the investigation and management of individuals with hereditary renal disorders.

Skeletal Disorders

Royce PM, Steinmann B (eds) (1993). *Connective Tissue and Its Heritable Disorders: Molecular Genetic and Medical Aspects.* New York: Wiley-Liss, 709 pp., cost ~$130

Any clinician working with individuals with connective tissue disorders should have ready access to this work authored by the experts in this field. A new edition should be available in 1999.

Also see Taybi and Lachman above under Detection of Fetal Anomalies by Ultrasound.

Skin

Spitz JL (1996) *Genodermatoses: A Full-Color Clinical Guide to Genetic Skin Disorders.* Baltimore: Williams & Wilkins, 338 pp., cost ~$90

A wonderfully graphic depiction of the major inherited skin disorders. Each condition is summarized in two pages with a schematic drawing of a person illustrating the primary findings on one page and a brief description of the key features, incidence, age of onset, differential diagnosis, laboratory data, management suggestions, and prognosis. "Clinical pearls" and suggestions for further reading are included.

Sybert VP (1997). *Genetic Skin Disorders.* New York: Oxford University Press, 675 pp., cost ~$246

Amazing color photographs, precise clinical descriptions, and information about treatment, prenatal diagnosis, inheritance, differential diagnoses, and patient support groups for an array of inherited skin disorders. I miss having incidence/prevalence figures but that is a minor complaint.

Cancer

Foulkes WD, Hodgson SV (eds) (1998). *Inherited Susceptibility to Cancer: Clinical, Predictive and Ethical Perspectives.* New York: Cambridge University Press, 350 pp., cost ~$85

A general overview of the hereditary contributions to cancer by site. The multiauthored discussions on the ethical, legal, and social issues of genetic testing and screening are thought-provoking.

Offit K (1998). *Clinical Cancer Genetics: Risk Counseling and Management.* New York: Wiley-Liss, 419 pp., cost ~$65 paper

A clinical overview of the various epidemiologic and hereditary factors involved in cancer. Emphasis is on the management of individuals with an increased risk to develop cancer as well as the many psychological, ethical, and legal issues in cancer risk counseling. This book is perfect for clinicians who want a good general overview of the field of cancer genetics. Those clinicians already practicing in the heart of this field may be left clamoring for more.

Schneider KA (1994). *Counseling About Cancer: Strategies for Genetic Counselors.* Available from the National Society of Genetic Counselors, 233 Canterbury Drive, Wallingford, PA 19086-6617, phone (610) 872-5959, pp. 147, cost ~$15.

This book is a classic in understanding some of the psychosocial and genetic counseling issues involved with genetic counseling for individuals with a family history of cancer. Unfortunately, this book is dated because it was published just before a myriad of new genetic tests became available for a variety of cancer susceptiblity gene alterations. A new edition is planned soon.

Vogelstein B, Kinzler KW (eds) (1998). *The Genetic Basis of Human Cancer.* New York: McGraw-Hill, 731 pp., cost ~$95, cloth

Vogelstein and Kinzler have brought together the experts in this field to provide a detailed look at the concepts in cancer genetics, the familial cancer syndromes, and site-specific cancers. The genetic counseling and ethical issues involved in cancer risk counseling are unfortunately missing from this volume. This book is a valuable resource for clinicians involved in the delivery of cancer genetics services, but may be more than is needed for the more general clinician who is looking for a good clinical overview on this topic.

Ethics

Andrews LB, Fullarton JE, Holtzman NA, Motulsky AG (eds) (1994). *Assessing Genetic Risks: Implications for Health and Social Policy.* Washington, DC: National Academy Press, 338 pp., cost ~$54

This report from the National Institute of Medicine of the National Academy of Sciences reviews important information about issues such as quality assurance in genetic testing; appropriate roles for public agencies, private health practitioners, research laboratories and centers, and companies involved in testing; the importance of genetic counseling for persons considering testing; and access to test results for insurance, employment, and other uses.

Clarke AJ (ed) (1998). *The Genetic Testing of Children.* BIOS Scientific Publishers, pp. 334, cost ~$135.

The first book to explore this important and controversial topic about the conflict between a parents right to know and the protection from harm when testing healthy children for genetic disorders.

Nelkin D, Lindee MS (1995). *The DNA Mystique: The Gene As A Cultural Icon.* New York: W. H. Freeman and Co., 276 pp., cost ~$13 paper

Patients are very concerned about the stigma of genetic disorders, and given the media hype around "genes" it is no wonder. The authors provide a fascinating analysis of how science and culture intersect to shape the social meaning of the gene.

Rothstein MA (ed) (1997). *Genetic Secrets: Protecting Privacy and Confidentiality in the Genetic Era.* New Haven and London: Yale University Press, 511 pp., cost ~$40

The authors explore the many contexts in which issues of genetic privacy arise, ranging from research and clinical setting, to the workplace, the patient–physician relationship, insurance issues, adoption, and educational and legal systems.

APPENDIX *A.6*

Genetics in Practice: Five Case Studies

CASE 1   NO NEWS IS GOOD NEWS: A FAMILY HISTORY OF MENTAL RETARDATION

Nathan, age 30 y, and his wife Natalie, age 28 y, are planning a pregnancy in the next year. They are concerned because Nathan's 36-year-old brother, Billy, is mildly mentally retarded.

The Medical-Family History

Records were obtained from Billy's evaluation for a seizure disorder at the Children's Hospital. He has an IQ of 60. He has no regression in his abilities. He lives with his parents. He is unable to make change or ride a bus independently. He is able to perform activities of daily living. Billy was the product of a full-term, nonstressed vaginal delivery. His mother did not take any medications during the pregnancy. She had an occasional glass of wine (perhaps 5 glasses total) during her pregnancy.

Billy is described as having an easy-going personality. He has no hearing or visual deficits. His speech is limited and repetitive. He is 5'10" tall. Because Billy lives on the other side of the country, it was not possible to examine him. Natalie and Nathan brought some of their wedding pictures to their appointment. Billy does not seem to have anything peculiar about the way he looks. His head appears normally shaped. His eyes and ears appear normally placed and shaped. He does not appear to have coarse facial features. His hair seems normal. His jaw appears somewhat prominent. Nathan does not recall any unusual birthmarks on his brother. Billy reportedly does not have any skeletal anomalies or joint laxity. He had multiple seizures beginning at age 3 years until the age of 19 years. He still takes a seizure

225

medication. His parents first noticed his delays soon after his seizures began. He does not appear to have any problems walking or with muscle weakness (several of the wedding pictures show him merrily joining in the dancing!). He has no involuntary movements. Billy is not described as having symptoms suggestive of a metabolic problem (Table 4.11), such as severe childhood illnesses, episodic vomiting, hypoglycemia, unusual odors, or an unusual dietary pattern. Nathan does not recall if his brother has large testes.

Billy is Nathan's only sibling. Their father, Nate, Sr., is 62 years old. He developed diabetes three years ago. His diabetes is under good control with medication. Nate had three older full siblings. Nate's oldest brother, Norman, died at age 70 years from a myocardial infarction. Norman and his wife had one miscarriage and two healthy daughters. Nate has two sisters—Edith, age 68 years, and Naomi, age 64 years. Edith has a son and a daughter who are both healthy. Naomi has a healthy son, Peter, from her first marriage, and a son, Carson, from her second marriage. Nate's father died of a heart attack at age 58 years. His mother is living at age 93 years. She has lost about 2 inches of height from osteoporosis, but is otherwise reasonably healthy.

Nathan and Billy's mother, JoAnne, age 63 years, had some knee surgery from a sports injury, but is otherwise healthy. She has two brothers—Roger, age 61 years, and a twin brother, Thomas. Roger has one daughter, and Thomas has three daughters and a son. They are all reportedly healthy. JoAnne's father died in a car accident at age 45 years, and her mother died at age 80 from pneumonia related to complications after a hip replacement.

JoAnne's father's family settled in the Ohio Valley more than 100 years ago; they were mostly of English and Irish ancestry. Her mother's father emigrated from Ireland in the early 1900s. Nathan laughs and states that his father's ancestry is "Heinz 57," although he is proud to say that his great-grandfather was a Native American from the Salish tribe.

Natalie is the youngest of eight siblings, having four full brothers and three full sisters. Her mother, Rosemary, is 76 years old and in good health. Natalie's father, Edward, had prostate cancer at age 75 years, but he is doing well at age 78 years. Edward came from a large family with three brothers and two sisters. They are all apparently healthy, as are their numerous children. Rosemary has a younger sister and a brother. Her sister never had children, and her brother has five healthy children. Rosemary's father and mother have lived in the United States for many years; their ancestors were mostly from Germany, France, and Holland. Edward's parents were also of Northern European ancestry.

Natalie and Nathan are not aware if their parents are related to each other either as cousins or more closely related. There is no other family history of mental retardation, birth defects, or miscarriages.

Pedigree Analysis

The most thorough approach to providing a risk assessment for Natalie and Nathan is to have Billy evaluated by a medical geneticist because the etiology of his developmental delay has never been determined. Initially, Natalie and Nathan were reluctant to pursue this option; they were concerned that Nathan's parents would feel guilty if they found out that Nathan and Natalie had a high chance to have a child with mental impairments. Nathan felt a conflict between his strong emotional attachment to Billy and his not wanting to have a child "like Billy." Nathan decided to approach his parents because he felt that a disease diagnosis for Billy might also benefit Billy's health and planning for his long-term care.

Nathan's parents agreed to have Billy evaluated by a medical geneticist near their home. A syndrome was not identified. Because Billy had never had a chromosome study or testing for fragile X syndrome, both of these studies were done. He also had plasma and urine amino acids, and urine organic acid analysis to rule out many of the common inborn errors of metabolism. These studies were normal.

The medical family history (Fig. A.1) does not provide any obvious indicators to a possible hereditary etiology to Billy's problems. It is possible to provide Nathan and Natalie with empirical risk figures to have a child with mental retardation based on their "normal" family history. The following risk possibilities were discussed with the couple:

1. Autosomal dominant inheritance seems unlikely because Nathan and his parents are of normal intelligence and they do not have any dysmorphic features. Billy could have a new dominant mutation but this would not affect his healthy adult brother.

2. Autosomal recessive inheritance is a possibility. If Billy's parents are related as cousins (or more closely related), the likelihood of autosomal recessive inheritance would be greater. Many inborn errors of metabolism are inherited in an autosomal recessive pattern (Table 4.11). Billy had normal studies of his plasma and urine amino acids, and urine organic acids, reducing but not eliminating the chances that he has an inborn error of metabolism.

3. If Billy's problems are a result of an autosomal recessive gene alteration, then Nathan's chance to be a heterozygous carrier is 2/3. Because Nathan and Natalie are not consanguineous, the chance that she also carries this same gene alteration is probably less than 1%. An estimate of their chance to have an affected child is 2/3 (Nathan's chance to carry the gene alteration) × 1/2 (the chance he passes the gene alteration to his child) × 1/100 (an estimated risk that Natalie is a carrier for the same autosomal recessive gene alteration) × 1/2 (the chance Natalie passes the gene alteration to her child) = 1/300.

4. Another possibility is that Billy's condition is X-linked. Fragile X syndrome is the most common form of mental retardation in males. Billy had a normal fragile X DNA test. Billy could still have some other form of X-linked mental retardation. JoAnne has two healthy brothers. This information does not rule out an X-linked syndrome, although it does slightly reduce the likelihood that Billy carries an X-linked gene mutation. Even if Billy did have an X-linked mutation, because Nathan is healthy, it is unlikely that he is harboring the same gene alteration.

5. A chromosome aberration should be considered in any individual with mental retardation. Billy's chromosome study was normal; therefore it is unlikely that Nathan carries a chromosome rearrangement.

6. Mitochondrial inheritance is an unlikely though remote possibility. Some mitochondrial disorders are associated with mental retardation and seizures. Given

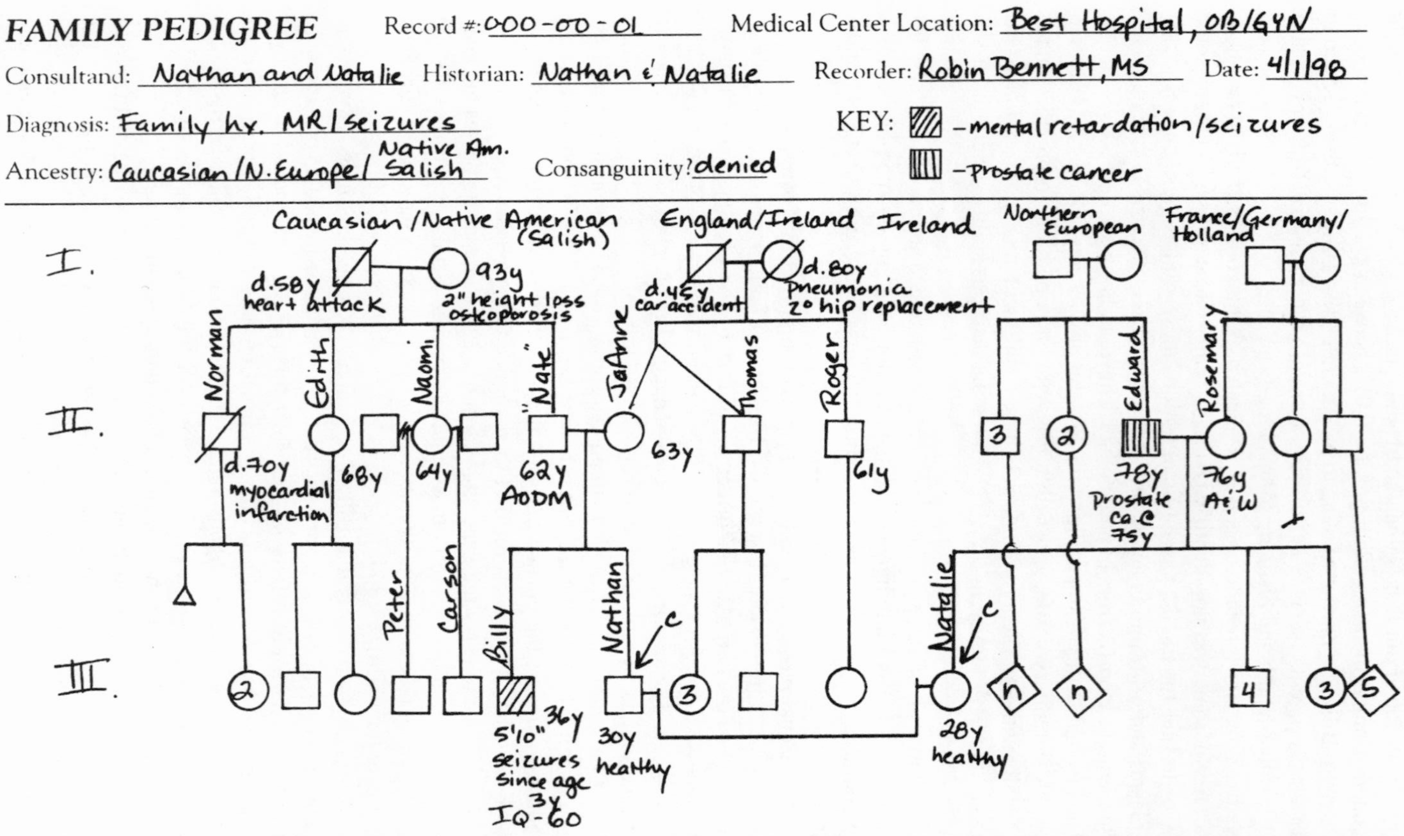

Figure A.1 Hypothetical pedigree of Nathan and Natalie. Nathan has a brother with an undiagnosed condition involving mental retardation and a seizure disorder.

that Billy's mother is apparently healthy, this is less likely. If this is a mitochondrial syndrome, Nathan does not appear to be affected, and Nathan's offspring would not be at risk because men do not pass mitochondria to their children.

In summary, the etiology of Billy's mental impairment remains unknown. His tests for the most likely causes of mental retardation (chromosomal imbalances and fragile X mutations) were negative. Given both Nathan and Natalie's noncontributory family histories, they can be given risk figures from empirical tables. The chance that a healthy sibling of a moderately retarded individual will have a similarly affected child is about 1.8%. This compares to the approximately 1% chance that any couple has to have a child with mental retardation.

Nathan and Natalie were reassured by this information. They have since gone on to have a healthy son and a healthy daughter.

CASE 2   A FRESH LOOK AT AN ADOLESCENT WITH CONGENITAL CATARACTS AND MENTAL RETARDATION

Bob Johnson is a 15-year-old moderately retarded youth who was found to have proteinuria when he was evaluated for his sports physical to participate in the Special Olympics. He was born blind, and he has had more than 20 surgeries for glaucoma and cataracts. His parents were told his congenital cataracts and mental retardation were a result of congenital rubella syndrome. Given the combination of congenital cataracts, mental retardation, and possible renal disease, it seemed wise to obtain a family history to see if there could be a genetic explanation for this combination of characteristics.

The Medical-Family History

Bob has proportionate short stature (height 134 cm, and weight 29 kg, both below the third percentile). His head circumference is 58.5 cm, which is above the 98th percentile. His blood pressure is 110/64. He has numerous sebaceous cysts on his face, hands, neck, buttocks, legs, and ears. His eyes are deep set and hypoteloric. He has a broad nasal root and broad nasal tip. He has a large mouth with full lips. His ears are large. His palate is normal. He is hirsute. His lungs are clear to auscultation. His heart has regular rate and rhythm. His abdomen is normal. He has normal male genitalia with bilateral descended testes. He has broad and short hands and feet. He has decreased range of motion and difficulty with ambulation, given joint stiffness particularly in his hips and knees. He does not have a history of diabetes or seizures.

Bob has quite a sense of humor and is very vocal. His mother, Ann, states he has some stereotypical behaviors such as head bumping and finger tapping. Ann is frustrated by Bob's disruptive temper tantrums. His development was delayed. Bob sat up at 2 years of age, walked at about age 2 1/2 years, developed his first words at 2 years, and was able to put a few words together by age 3 1/2 years. He can sign his name. Bob does not have regression of his learning.

Ann did have a fever and joint aches early in her pregnancy. She did not consume any alcohol or drugs during her pregnancy. Bob was delivered vaginally at 40 weeks gestation. His cataracts were noted a few days after birth. Ann was told by Bob's pediatrician that the rubella she had had while pregnant was the cause of Bob's problems.

Bob has a healthy sister, Julie, age 19 years. Julie attends college in a premedical curriculum. Julie is 5'6 " tall and has no health problems. Bob's mother, Ann, is 47 years old and is employed as an accountant. She has recently been diagnosed with cataracts. She is otherwise healthy. She had a brother, John, who died at age 37 years. Ann is not sure of the cause of her brother's death; he grew up in a home for the learning disabled. He had severe mental retardation, glaucoma, and cataracts. Ann's mother, Sophie, died last year at age 77 years. She was recovering from a hip replacement and died of pneumonia. Sophie had one sister, Jasmine, who is reportedly healthy at age 75 years. She had one daughter, Georgia, who is healthy at age 45 years. Ann has little contact with this distant branch of the family, but apparently Georgia's youngest son, Sam, has cataracts, glaucoma, and some developmental disabilities. Ann believes Sam is about 12 years old and that he has two healthy sisters in middle-school.

Bob's mother and father (Jim) divorced when Bob was 5 years old. Jim has not remained in contact with the family. Ann believes Jim has at least two other sons. Ann is not aware of any health problems in Jim or his sons. Jim came from a large family of three sisters and two brothers. Ann believes that they are all healthy as are their children. Ann knows that her ex-husband's parents are deceased but she is not sure of the causes. Jim is 48 years old and is 5'11" tall.

Jim and Ann are both of African American ancestry. They are not known to be consanguineous.

Pedigree Analysis

It is unlikely that Bob, John, and Sam have glaucoma, cataracts, and varying degrees of mental retardation by chance alone. The most likely explanation is an X-linked inheritance pattern because the affected males are related through apparently healthy women. Ann's early cataracts are probably a manifestation of her being heterozygous for the gene alteration. It might be possible to obtain the prenatal records from Ann's pregnancy with Bob to document the occurrence of maternal rubella. Usually children with congenital rubella have small heads, and Bob has a large head. A syndrome with autosomal dominant inheritance with reduced penetrance is a possibility but less likely because predominantly males are affected, and the only female who is possibly affected (Ann) has mild manifestations in comparison to the male relatives. The family could have an inherited chromosomal translocation where by chance only males have been affected. No one in the family is known to have had a miscarriage. Mitochondrial inheritance is another possibility because the males are affected through females. However, you would expect to see females who are as severely affected as males. Progression of the disease is often seen in mitochondrial disorders (owing to a continuing accumulation of mitochondrial mutations during cell division); there does not seem to be progression of the disease in Bob.

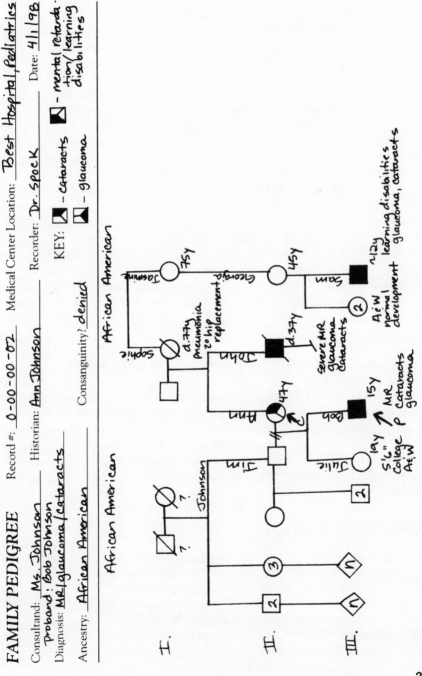

Figure A.2 *Hypothetical pedigree of the Johnson family—a family with X-linked oculocerebrorenal (Lowe) syndrome.*

The collection of characteristics of congenital cataracts, mental retardation, short stature, sebaceous cysts, dysmorphic features, joint problems, and probable renal disease (Fig. A.2) is suggestive of the X-linked oculocerebrorenal (Lowe) syndrome (Table 4.9). A medical geneticist, using the appropriate diagnostic testing, confirmed this diagnosis in Bob. Because progressive tubular and glomerular renal disease is a major component of the syndrome, Bob was referred for a full assessment of his renal function. Treatment with phosphorus, calcium, carnitine, and/or vitamin D is usually beneficial for these individuals in managing their renal disease and bone degeneration.

Multiple family members were affected by a fresh look at Bob's medical-family history. Ann was pleased she finally had an explanation for her son's problems. She had always felt guilty that her son's problems were a result of something she had done in the pregnancy. Knowledge that her son's temper outbursts were characteristic of boys with this condition was a relief because Ann had fretted that her parenting techniques were at fault. Ann was grateful to learn of the national support group for families with Lowe syndrome (the Lowe Foundation), and she could hardly wait to attend their next annual meeting to meet other parents who had children with similar problems. Ann planned to share information about Lowe syndrome with her daughter, who has a 50:50 chance to be a carrier of the oculocerebrorenal syndrome, so that Julie can make her own choices about childbearing and prenatal testing. Because Lowe syndrome is a multi-system disease, a final diagnosis in Bob is beneficial for his life-long health management. Sharing this information with Sam's parents and health-care providers will also assist in his medical care.

CASE 3 BUT I THOUGHT THAT WAS A PEDIATRIC DISEASE . . .

Mrs. Rhonda Adams is a 40 year-old Caucasian woman seeking a new primary care physician because she has recently moved to this area. She has been successful in her career as a computer programmer for the past 15 years. She has a significant history of chronic respiratory disease. She is a nonsmoker and nobody smokes in her household. As a child she had chronic sinusitis, and she has been hospitalized several times for pneumonia. She has constant postnasal drip. She has intermittent heartburn.

The Medical-Family History

Rhonda and her husband Ron have two healthy children—A daughter Jane, age 20 years, and a daughter, Angie, age 18 years. Mrs. Adams has three full siblings. Her sister, Frieda, is 45 years old and has two healthy sons, ages 22 and 17. A sister, Stephanie, is 43 years old. She has nasal polyps and had one miscarriage at approximately 12 weeks gestation. A brother, Paul, is 36 years old. He and his wife have been trying to conceive a pregnancy for about 3 years. They have an appointment to see a fertility specialist.

Mrs. Adam's mother, Joyce, died at age 65 from a myocardial infarction. She had one brother who died at age 24 in World War II. A sister is healthy at age 68 years, as are her three children and eight grandchildren. Joyce's mother died at age 85 of colon cancer, and Joyce's father died at age 77 of "old age." They are of Russian–German (Ashkenazi Jewish) ancestry.

Mrs. Adam's father, Robert, has some arthritis at age 75 but is otherwise healthy. He has two older sisters, ages 78 and 80 years, who are reportedly healthy, as are their children. A full sister died in infancy of unknown causes. Robert's father died of heart disease at age 90. Robert's mother had Parkinson's disease and died in her 80s. They are of Polish (Ashkenazi Jewish) ancestry. The families are not known to be consanguineous.

There is no other history of miscarriages, infertility, or deaths in childhood. There is no family history of liver or pancreatic dysfunction or gastrointestinal disease. Mrs. Adams does not report having foul smelling stools although she describes her stomach as always being a little "sensitive."

Pedigree Analysis

The family history is suggestive of cystic fibrosis (Fig. A.3). Paul's infertility could be due to congenital absence of the vas deferens. The report of nasal polyps in Stefanie and problems conceiving a pregnancy is also suggestive of cystic fibrosis. The family history is compatible with autosomal recessive inheritance because there does not appear to be related health problems in more than one generation.

Mrs. Adams was referred for a genetic evaluation, including a sweat-chloride test and DNA mutation analysis for mutations in the cystic fibrosis gene. Her sweat chloride was abnormal. She is a compound heterozygote for two of the more common mutations in the Caucasian/Northern European population—delta F508 and R117H.

Mrs. Adam's diagnosis of cystic fibrosis will now assist in the management of her pulmonary disease. Her siblings may have minor pulmonary manifestations of cystic fibrosis. Knowing whether or not they have cystic fibrosis can be important in their health care. The diagnosis of affected or carrier status can be determined with DNA testing. Paul most likely has congenital absence of the vas deferns (see Section 4.16). At age 43, Stephanie may be considering future pregnancies. Decreased fertility in women is associated with cystic fibrosis. If Stephanie has inherited one or both mutations, her husband may want to have cystic fibrosis carrier testing. Mrs. Adam's daughters are obligate carriers for a cystic fibrosis mutation. This information is important for their own family planning.

CASE 4   LIFE ISN'T ALWAYS AS IT SEEMS

Jill is a successful 40-year-old costume designer for a local theater group. She is petrified of the cancer that she describes as "running rampant" in her family. This

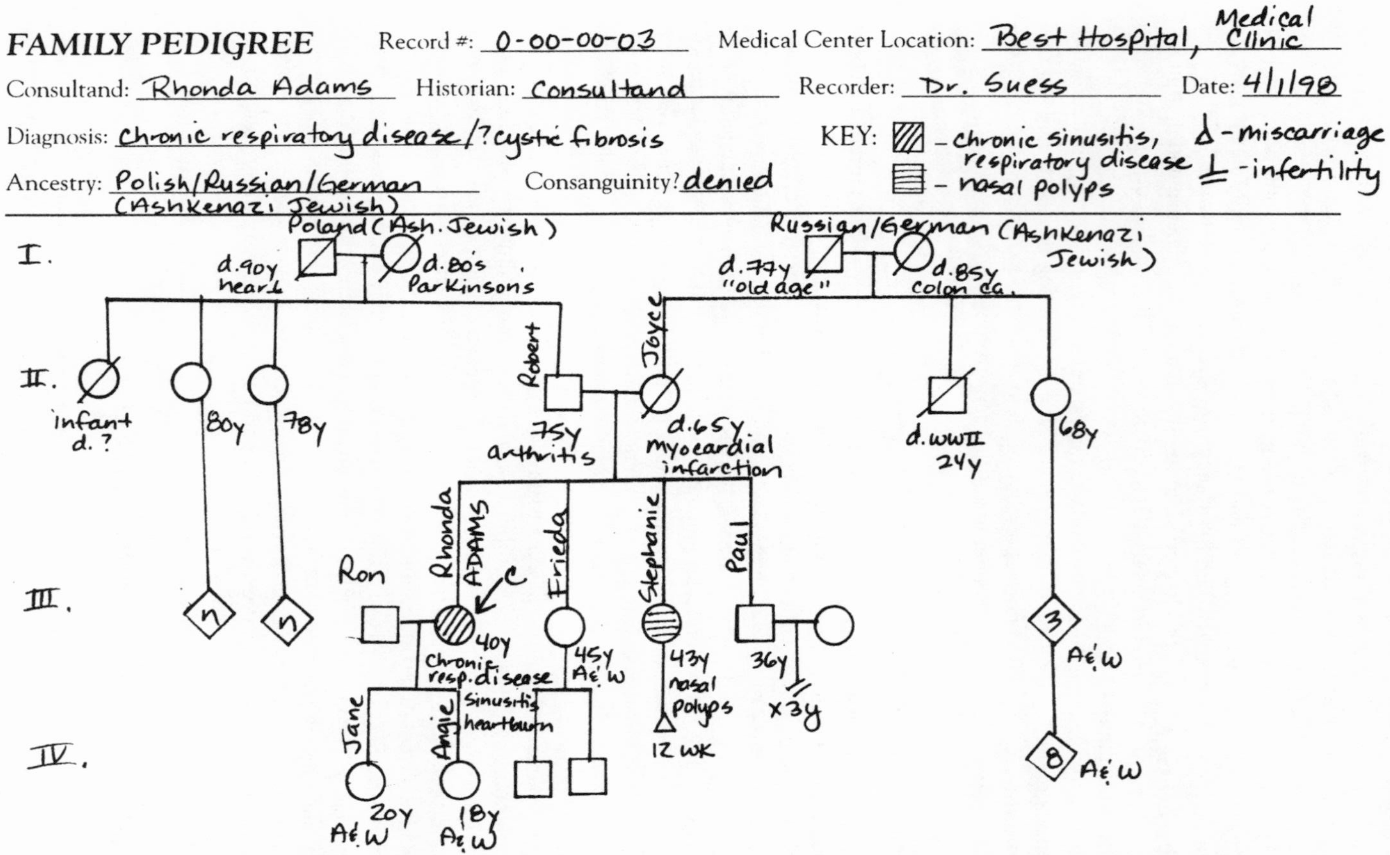

234

FAMILY PEDIGREE   Record #: 0-00-00-03   Medical Center Location: Best Hospital, Medical Clinic

Consultand: Rhonda Adams   Historian: Consultand   Recorder: Dr. Suess   Date: 4/1/98

Diagnosis: chronic respiratory disease/? cystic fibrosis

Ancestry: Polish/Russian/German (Ashkenazi Jewish)

Consanguinity? denied

KEY: ▨ – chronic sinusitis, respiratory disease, nasal polyps   ▤ – ⸗   δ – miscarriage   ⊥ – infertility

(pedigree diagram with labels: d.90y heart, d.80s Parkinsons, Poland (Ash. Jewish), Russian/German, d.74y "old age", Russian/German (Ashkenazi Jewish), d.85y colon ca, 68y, d.WWII 24y, 3 A&W, 8 A&W, infant d.?, 80y, 78y, 5, 5, Robert, 75y arthritis, d.65y myocardial infarction, 76y ca, Paul, 36y, Rex, Stephanie 43y nasal polyps 12 wk, Frieda 45y A&W, Rhonda ADAMS 40y chronic resp. disease sinusitis, Ron, Angie 18y A&W heartburn, Jane 20y A&W)

Figure A.3 Hypothetical pedigree of Rhonda Adams—a woman with chronic respiratory disease who has cystic fibrosis.

visit is prompted by the recent diagnosis of prostate cancer in her 76-year-old father, Thomas. Jill is considering having a prophylactic oophorectomy. Her mother, Evelyn, died 30 years ago of ovarian cancer at the age 44 years. Jill has heard that breast and ovarian cancer can "run in a family." She states "Since I'm through having children, I would consider both having my breasts and ovaries removed if this will allow me to live to watch my children grow old."

Medical-Family History

Jill and her partner Dan have two daughters, ages six years and 15 months. Jill is the only child of her mother and father, although she has two healthy half brothers from her father's first marriage: Patrick, age 48 years, and Samuel, age 50 years. Samuel has two healthy children, ages 30 and 27 years. Patrick has never had biological children but has two healthy step daughters. Dan is of Mexican-American ancestry and he and Jill are not blood relatives.

Jill knows little about her mother's treatment for cancer. She knows her mother was diagnosed with cancer about a year before she died. Jill believes her mother was trying to "protect her." Jill is tearful as she recalls her mother's death. She recalls her mother as being a gracious hostess and fabulous actress, although Jill regrets that her mother "enjoyed her Vodka Collins" and "smoked like a chimney" until her death. Evelyn was estranged from her family because her parents were apparently upset with her choice of "a life in the world of theater," and because Evelyn died when Jill was only 10 years old, Jill knows little of her mother's medical-family history. According to Jill, Evelyn left home at the age of 17 years because she found it difficult to live in an alcoholic home with a verbally abusive father. Jill believes her mother's brother, Clark, died in his 50s from stomach cancer. He had no children. Jill is in contact with her mother's sister, Betty, who is apparently healthy at age 75 years. Betty has a son, Mark, age 45 years, and a daughter, Judy, age 48 years. Jill and Judy see each other socially quite often, and Judy recently confided in Jill that she had an abnormal Pap smear. Evelyn had another brother, Jack, who died of unknown kidney problems at age 67. He had at least three children but Jill does not even know their names. Evelyn's mother, Janis, apparently died of brain cancer at the age of 78 years, and Evelyn's father, Bradley, committed suicide at the age of 60 years. He apparently was an alcoholic. Evelyn's parents met in their early 20s when they both were working in a textile factory in New York City. Both Evelyn's mother and father emigrated from England.

Jill's father, Thomas, is a retired attorney. He has one sister, Deidra, who is 70 years old and has one healthy daughter. Another sister, Janet, has heart disease at age 63 but is otherwise healthy. Janet has a son and a daughter. Thomas grew up in Alaska and is of Native American (Tlingit tribe) ancestry. Thomas and Evelyn were divorced when Jill was only 2 years old, and Jill went to live with her father after her mother's death. His father died of "old age" at the age of 80 years, and his mother is alive at age 97 years!

Pedigree Analysis

On the surface there seems to be a lot of cancer in this family which may represent a familial cancer syndrome (Fig. A.4). To be absolutely certain, it is essential to obtain medical records and death certificates on the family members with cancer. With the help of Jill's aunt Betty, Jill is able to obtain the pathology reports on her mother's cancer diagnosis, and death certificates on her uncle and maternal grandmother. Evelyn's medical records indicate that actually Evelyn had a metastatic abdominal cancer of unknown primary origin, but the surgical report indicates that the ovaries looked healthy. Jill and her aunt requested Clark's death certificate because they were unsure where he had his medical care. According to the death certificate, Clark died at age 64 years from metastatic melanoma. Jill's aunt Betty also adds to this history that her brothers and sister, and their father, had problems with alcohol abuse, and the whole family smoked heavily. Jack died of renal failure related to complications from diabetes and alcohol abuse. Evelyn's mother's death certificate states she died of metastatic brain cancer from the bladder.

Jill's family may have a single gene mutation or mutations in more than one gene that predispose to cancer susceptibility (particularly if exposed to strong carcinogenic agents such as tobacco smoke). The occurrence of brain cancer in Jill's maternal grandmother Janis is probably explained by environmental factors, not heredity; bladder cancer is one of the most common cancers seen in heavy smokers, and brain cancer is a known metastatic site for bladder cancer (see Tables 5.5 and 5.6). Janis may have also been exposed to carcinogenic agents in the textile factory she was working at in the early 1900s. Aunt Betty also told Jill that Jill's uncles were notoriously noncompliant with their health care because they were reluctant to "give up their cigarettes and martinis."

Given that Jill has multiple relatives with cancer, she should be judicious with her cancer screening, but her family history does not suggest that she needs to have screening at ages or intervals different from any other woman her age. Given her strong family history of alcohol abuse, she would be wise to use alcohol in moderation.

Jill was thrilled with this information. She thought that her family history was a "cancer death sentence." As Jill approached the age that her mother had died, her fear of ovarian cancer becoming overwhelming; from all her research, Jill felt the prognosis for anyone given a diagnosis of ovarian cancer was grim. She was greatly comforted that her mother's cancer was probably not ovarian in origin, and indeed may have been related to her smoking and alcohol use. Jill was aware that she has no guarantees that she does not have an increased risk for cancer, but she does not need to be screened for cancer any differently from other women her age. Although obtaining information about Jill's family was time consuming it helped Jill obtain peace of mind and saved her from further debate over the consideration of a prophylactic oophorectomy.

FAMILY PEDIGREE

Record #: 0-00-60-04   Medical Center Location: Best Hospital

Consultand: Jill   Historian: Same   Recorder: Dr. M. Horton   Date: 4/1/98

Diagnosis: family hx cancer (melanoma, bladder)

Ancestry: Native American/England   Consanguinity? denied

KEY: ☐ - melanoma   ◪ - prostate ca.
     ☐ - bladder ca.   ⊘ - metastatic ca. unknown primary

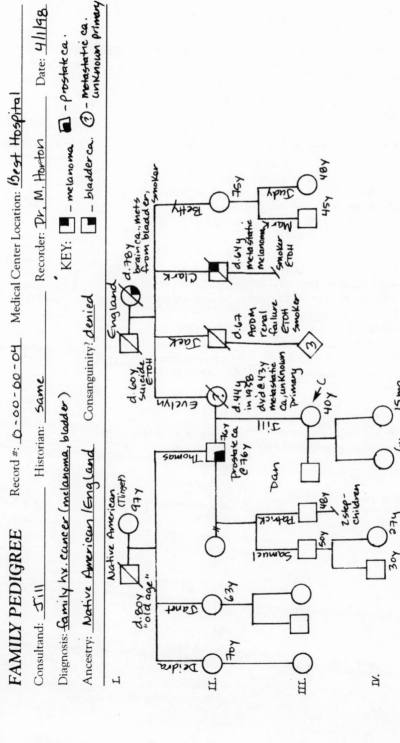

Figure A.4   Hypothetical pedigree of Jill—a woman with a family history of cancer.

237

CASE 5 A PEDIGREE PICKLE

I like to use this song for a fun break in teaching (Fig. A.5).

I'm My Own Grandpaw. Words and Music by Dwight Latham and Moe Jaffe © 1947 (renewed 1975) COLGEMS-EMI MUSIC INC. All Rights Reserved International Copyright Secured Used by Permission.

Many, many years ago when I was twenty-three
I was married to a widow who was pretty as could be.
This widow had a grown up daughter who had hair of red.
My father fell in love with her and soon, they too, were wed.
   Chorus
This made my dad my son-in-law, and changed my very life.
For my daughter was my mother cause she was my father's wife.
To complicate the matter even though it brought me joy,
I soon became the father of a bouncing baby boy.
   Chorus
My little baby then became a brother-in-law to Dad,
And so became my uncle, though it made me very sad.
For if he was my uncle then that also made him brother
Of the widow's grown-up daughter who, of course, was my stepmother.
   Chorus
Father's wife then had a son who kept them on the run.
And he became my grandchild for he was my daughter's son.
My wife is now my mother's mother and it makes me blue
Because, although she is my wife, she's my gradmother too.
   Chorus
Oh, if my wife is my grandmother, then I am her grandchild
And everytime I think of it it nearly drives me wild.
For now I have become the strangest case you ever saw;
As husband of my grandmother I am my own grandpaw.

Chorus
I'm my own grandpaw.
I'm my own grandpaw.
It sounds funny, I know,
But it really is so;
I'm my own grandpaw.

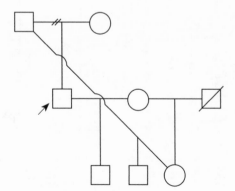

Figure A.5 *Teaching tool: Pedigree of a man who is his own grandfather.*

Index

Skeletal disorders
  cubitis valgus, 75
  dysplasias, 117–118
  hearing loss and, 87
  questions to ask about, generally, 57
  pectus carinatum, 75
  pectus excavatum, 75
  short stature anomalies and disorders, 26,
    115–119
Skin disorders
  café au lait spots, 75, 98, 130
  hypopigmentation, 75
  questions to ask about, 57, 98
Skin cancer, 132–133, 135–136, 138–139
Slater, Eliot, 13
Smith-Lemli-Opitz syndrome, 22, 73, 75, 90–91,
    115–117
Software
  family history data, 152
  pedigree drawing, 212–213
Somatic mosaicism, 34
Sperm donation, 160–164
Spina bifida, 77. *See also* Neural tube defects
Spinal muscular atrophy, 22
Spinobulbar muscular atrophy, 28, 102, 121
Spinocerebellar ataxias, 28, 99, 105
Spondyloepiphyseal dysplasia congenita, 117
Spontaneous abortion, symbol, 47
Sporadic conditions, 34
Sporadic inheritance, 13–14
SRY gene, 25
Steroid sulfatase deficiency, 121
Stickler syndrome, 91
Stigmatization, genetic disorders and, 54, 106,
    167
Stillbirth, 47, 214
Storage disorders, 102
Stroke, 31
Sudden infant death syndrome (SIDS), 123–124
Support groups, patient genetic disease, 213
Surrogacy, pedigree symbols, 163–164
Survivor guilt, 170
Susceptibility genetic testing, 52
Symbols, pedigree
  adoption, 49–50
  affected status, 46, 50
  A&W, 50
  blended families, 45, 47
  consultand, 46
  deceased, 46
  family hearsay, 50
  family history unknown, 50
  females, 46
  gamete donation, 163–164

  infertility, 47, 50
  miscarriage (SAB), 27,
  multiple partners, 47
  no children by choice, 47, 50
  pregnancy and reproduction-related, 45–47
  proband, 46
  sex unknown, 46
  siblings, 42, 45
  surrogacy, 163–164
  termination of pregnancy (TOP), 47
  test results, 53
  twins, 42
Syndactyly, 76
Syndromic deafness, 83
Syphilis, 104, 107, 116
Systemic disease 107
Systemic lupus erythematosus, 80, 108

Taylor, Elizabeth, 48
Tay-Sachs disease, 7–8, 20, 22, 106, 107
Teeth anomalies, 74, 86
Teratogens, implications of
  cardiac, 80
  environmental teratogens, 71, 87
  generally, 120
  human, 60
  minor anomalies and, 73–75
Termination of pregnancy (TOP), symbol, 47
Testicular feminization, 121
Testing, types of
  diagnostic, 95
  DNA, 17, 61, 154
  genetic, generally, 52, 140–142, 157–158
  metabolic, 104
  molecular genetic blood, 100
  ophthalmologic, 104
  paternity, 17
  predictive, 54
  prenatal, 169
Thalassemia, beta, 22
Therapeutic donor insemination, 160–164
Third-degree relatives, 43–44
Threatening, genetic disorders as, 167–168
Thymine (T), 14
Thyroid
  carcinoma, 131–135
  disease, 131, 133
Tobacco use
  cancer, 129, 139
  maternal and orofacial clefting, 79
  miscarriage and maternal, 120
  respiratory disease and, 112
Tonic-clonic seizures, 102
Toxoplasmosis, 89, 103, 116

Transcription, 14
Translation, 14
Treacher-Collins syndrome. *See* Mandibulofacial dysostosis
Trichorhinophalangeal syndrome (TRPS), 74, 86
Trimethadione, fetal, 80, 114, 116
Trinucleotide repeat disorders, 13, 27–28, 104
Triplet repeat disorders. *See* Trinucleotide repeat disorders
Trisomy 13, 73–75, 77, 116, 118
Trisomy 18, 27, 73–75, 77, 116, 118
Trisomy 21 (Down syndrome), 26–27, 34, 69, 71–75
Truth, in pedigree, 173–174
Tuberous sclerosis complex
 autism and, 99
 gene locus, 132
 growths/tumors in, 135
 hamartomas, retinal, 135
 hypopigmentation, skin 75
 kidney disease in, 113–115
 learning disabilities and mental retardation in, 98,135
 malignancies, 135
 prevalence, 20
 seizures in, 103
Tubular disorders, of renal system, 13
Tumors, benign, 133–134
Turcot syndrome, 134
Turner syndrome, 27, 73, 75, 110, 116, 118, 120
Twins
 major depression, research study, 108
 in pedigree, 42
Tyrosinemia, 114

Ultrasound
 fetal anomalies, detection by, 81–82
 information resources, 221
 medical-family history questions for abnormal, 82
Uniparental disomy (UPD), 33
Unpatient, defined, 168
Unremarkable family history, 63, 65
Uremic syndromes, 107, 113
Urinary tract, malformation of, 112
Usher syndrome, 22, 86
Uterine cancer, 133, 138

Valproate syndrome, fetal, 74–75, 80–81

Van der Woude syndrome, 20, 74, 79, 86
Variable expression, 17–18
Varicella, fetal, 89, 91, 116
Vascular disease, 104
Vas deferens, congenital absence of, 121–122
Velocardiofacial syndrome (VCFS)
 cleft palate, 79
 congenital heart defects, 80
 minor anomalies, 74
 schizophrenic-like symptoms, 98, 107
Visual disorders, 88–92
VitalChek Network, Inc., 150
Vitamin B_{12} defciency, 107
Vomiting, episodic, 93, 97
Von Hippel-Lindau (VHL) syndrome, 5–7, 9–10, 13, 20, 113–114, 130–132

Waardenburg syndrome, 20, 73, 75, 86
Warburg syndrome, 90
Warfarin, 116
Werner syndrome, 91, 136
Wertz, Dorothy, Dr., 158
Wexler, Nancy, Dr., 177
Williams syndrome, 74–75, 116
Williams, Terry Tempest, 129
Wilms' tumor syndrome, 114–115, 130–132, 136
Wilson disease, 90, 107–109, 113–115
Wolfram syndrome, 119
Word choice, importance of, 54–55. *See also* Interviews
World of Genetics Societies, 171

X chromosome, 14
Xeroderma pigmentosum, 116–136
X-inactivation, 21
X-linked dominant (XLD) inheritance, 15–16
X-linked inheritance
 dominant, 23
 recessive (XLR), 16, 21, 23–25
X-linked mental retardation, 92
X-linked recessive inheritance, 15
XXX syndrome, 120

Y chromosome, 14
Y-deletions, implications of, 121–122
Y-linked inheritance (holandric), 16–25
Young syndrome, 11–112, 121–123

Zellweger syndrome, 90, 113, 115